CAN
No, Not Me!

by
Roseann Gallagher

J.A.G. Books Ltd

First published by J.A.G. Books Ltd 2010

Copyright © Roseann Gallagher 2010

All rights reserved. No part of this publication may be reproduced, stored in a retrieval system or transmitted in any form or by any means, electronic, mechanical, audio, visual or otherwise, without prior written permission of the copyright owner. Nor can it be circulated in any form of binding or cover other than that in which it is published and without similar conditions including this condition being imposed on the subsequent purchaser.

ISBN 978-0-9567708-0-6

Cover design by The Caley Group

http://caleyprint.com

Edited by Jan Andersen

http://www.creativecopywriter.org

J.A.G. Books Ltd
77 Farmington Avenue
Glasgow
G32 0BJ

Dedication

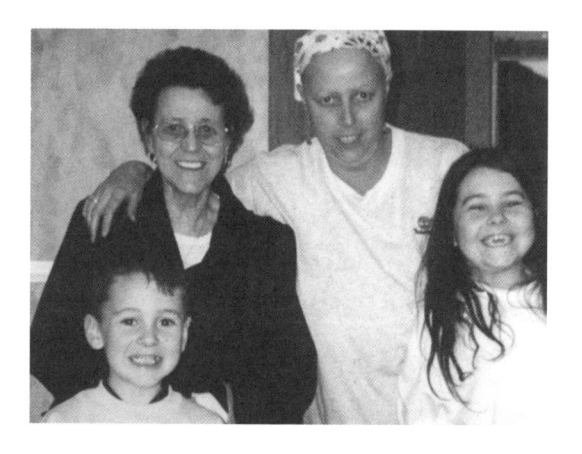

MUM

To you I solely dedicate this book, for without your inspiration I would never have found the strength, courage or belief in myself to put pen to paper in my quest to share such intimate, unspoken and personal experiences with others.

You wiped my tears in moments of despair, gave me hope when I felt weak and love when I felt lost.

Taken from us so suddenly, we have a void in our hearts that is only comforted by knowing that you are watching over us and a day will come when again we can embrace.

Annie Young
Feburary 1936 – May 2003

Acknowledgements

I would like to express a huge heartfelt thank you to Professor Cooke, Alison, Jean, Isabell and Marie. You are all true credits to your professions as well as exceptional individuals.

To all others touched by cancer who shared in my journey as I shared in theirs. My life has been uplifted at having crossed your paths in life.

To my friends and neighbours who supported me in so many ways; I thank you all.

To my wonderful sisters; thank you for your love and understanding when faced with a very difficult period in all our lives.

To my Mum and Dad; I love you.

To my wonderful son Billy and granddaughters Rebecca and Nicola; the goals I set, however small, were to reach periods in your lives of which I needed so desperately to be a part. Setting them made me strong. I am humbled by the gift of life to remain here with you.

To my wonderful editor, Jan Andersen; not only did you professionally support me as my editor, but truly felt my emotional and physical experiences as if your own. My life has been touched by the crossing of our paths, which has flourished into an ongoing road of kindred spirits and friendship.

I would also like to thank Craig Lind and Caleyprint for their input in both the cover design and printing of my book.

To Shahida of Perfect Publishers Limited thank you for co-ordinating an excellent team of professionals to produce the finished product that is now my book.

Last, but not least, to John, my wonderful husband and soul mate; if ever I doubted myself, you embraced me with love and made me believe I could move mountains. You understood my very being and the soul within me. Without you by my side and embracing my despair as one, I could not have travelled this voyage. You made me proud of the woman I became. Life is so cruel to have taken you from me, but destiny lies before us on another plane.

Disclaimer

All personal events contained within this book are true. However, some names have been changed or omitted to protect the identities of those concerned.

I, the author of this book, am committed to protecting the privacy of those mentioned within the book. I do not take legal responsibility if anyone mentioned within the book, or if any other individual voluntarily chooses to reveal the identity of the individuals mentioned in the book to the media or otherwise. In addition, any outside source, whether an individual or media source, takes full responsibility for the accuracy, timeliness and nature of anything said or published following the publication of this book. I, the author of this book, do not take responsibility for anything said, claimed or published by a third party following the publication of this book.

No material from this book may be copied, reproduced, republished, uploaded, posted, transmitted, quoted, or distributed in any way without the express permission of the author of this book.

Contents

    Preface. viii

1. Life 1
2. Realising the Truth 20
3. A Maze of Muddle 40
4. Reality. 49
5. It Was Time. 67
6. Struggling 77
7. Swings and Roundabouts 95
8. Will I Ever Get Out of Here?. 130
9. Home at Last. 137
10. Out, In, Out 150
11. The Run Up. 160
12. Chemotherapy: I'm Ready 173
13. It's Good to Laugh and be Blessed by Friends 199
14. Let's Start Round Two. 205
15. Benefits, Bills and People We Meet 211
16. He was Nice and They were Awful. 218
17. I'm a Poet and I Didn't Know It 223
18. Back to the Grind 227
19. It Was a Privilege to Call Her my Friend. 243
20. Time for a Radiotherapy Sun Tan. 248
21. Hi, My Name's Roseann 281

    I Am Not Alone. 285
    Epilogue 287

Preface

YES, ME.

I have written this book primarily to share my experiences, doubts, hopes and fears with the many individuals who, like me, find themselves facing this most daunting illness.

In addition, I hope to help professionals, families and friends of cancer sufferers gain an understanding and an insight into how cancer affects the individual who has, or has had cancer; a topic that to this day is still relatively taboo.

Strangely, no matter what form or type of cancer with which one is diagnosed, I have found through my own experience that when meeting others who have also come face to face with this terrible disease, we seem automatically to share this great unseen respect for each other, which at times can be totally overwhelming.

An elite club we surely are.

Chapter One

Life

How did it begin; this road I found myself going down? Well, like the majority of people I was sailing along quite happily with my life. I worked full-time as an assistant manager in Care Housing for frail elderly people, an area I might add in which I had been working for the previous twenty years and which I loved. I also worked in the voluntary sector as an advocate in the West End of town.

I had a lovely home, which I shared with my husband John, son Billy and my dog (my baby) Tess. I also had the advantage of coming from a very large, close knit family. My father and mother were very much alive and kicking and I had four lovely sisters, Issy, Iris, Janet and Debbie.

I also had two lovely grandchildren, Rebecca and Nicola, Billy's daughters from a long term relationship that had broken up some years prior. The girls were my pride and joy. They were a major part of our lives and visited most weekends. Life in my eyes was going well.

A big bonus, although I didn't realise it at the time, was that we all lived within a one mile radius of each other, with the exception of my sister Janet who lived down south.

Working full-time, as well as on a voluntary basis and performing all the other little tasks that seem to engulf our everyday lives, all contributed to the fact that I didn't really take as much time as I should have to be with my family. Like many people I would genuinely intend to, but there was always something or other that I would get caught up in that would eventually lead to me cancelling a visit to see my mum and dad, or one of my sisters. Before I even knew it, maybe a month would have passed and I had still not seen them. It was a standing joke of my dad's to shout out as I walked through the living-room door of his house, "Oh hello stranger; who are you?" This would then lead to me providing a whole list of excuses as to why I had not been down to visit. On leaving I would promise to visit more often, but I never got around to it.

John and I had always dreamed of going on a holiday of a lifetime to America, not the usual sightseeing holiday to Disneyland, but to travel to both Las Vegas and Los Angeles. It was our dream to take a helicopter ride into the Grand Canyon and to visit Beverly Hills. "Let's face it", we would say to each other, "you only live once". We knew that it wouldn't be cheap, but we were determined to go. It was September 1999 and this inevitably meant that both John and I would have to work overtime to help fund our adventure.

When I think back to that time, I must admit that I did remember feeling constantly tired! However, I dismissed this as being largely due to the extra workload I had taken on. I never gave a thought to the fact that my life consisted only of work and sleep and not much else. I shrugged off my feelings of exhaustion, telling myself that it would all be worth it in the end. So, I plodded on regardless, focusing only on the rewards of all my hard work; our dream holiday to America.

A few months prior to this, however, I had been taking a bath and whilst drying myself I noticed that the nipple on my left breast had become slightly inverted. However, I felt that I had no cause to be concerned because no sooner had the change taken place, than it would just as quickly rectify itself. Giving myself a quick breast examination, I could feel nothing out of the ordinary so continued drying my body, pushing the incident to the back of my mind. Time went by and all recollection of this experience had been forgotten, that is until the same thing happened. "Strange," I thought, "Best keep an eye on it just to be on the safe side".

Again, time went by and with no other signs or symptoms of anything untoward, I went on regardless, putting my problem down to the weight of my rather ample breasts being the culprit for the noted changes to my nipple.

One day, I visited my doctor's surgery for Hormone Replacement Therapy, which I required due to the fact that four years previously I had undergone a full hysterectomy. The female doctor that was seeing me that day looked rather perplexed as she commented on my left nipple being inverted, whilst giving me a routine breast examination. On explaining that I was fully aware of these changes, I then went on to inform her that I had been monitoring the situation and could find nothing wrong; no lumps or bumps that might have signified an underlying problem. After completing another, but more in-depth breast examination, the doctor informed me that she could also detect no abnormalities. I left the surgery feeling unconcerned.

As the weeks passed, I carried on regardless, even though it had now become apparent that my left nipple was inverted more often than not. However, after being nagged constantly by my husband John to have another check-up, I reluctantly made another appointment to visit my doctor's surgery, just to be on the safe side.

This time I saw a different female doctor at the practice, so there I was again explaining exactly what had been going on since I initially noticed the change in my left nipple and also the outcome of my previous visit to the surgery. This doctor, like the last, gave me a full breast examination and on finding nothing else apparently wrong, told me that with no other signs and symptoms she also was unable to pinpoint what could be causing my nipple to invert. I did enquire at this point if the doctor felt that there was a possibility that I could have breast cancer. Looking unconcerned, but without really giving me a direct answer, the doctor informed me that it was important that I continue to monitor my breasts, emphasising that should I note any further changes, I should make another appointment to see her or one of the other doctors at the practice.

Leaving the surgery, I mulled over in my head what had gone on during my consultation. Although I thought the doctor had been reluctant to answer my question as to whether I could have breast cancer, she had not been overly concerned about the problems that I had been experiencing and because of that, I returned home confident in my own belief that there was nothing to worry about. On John's return home from work that day, I firmly reassured him also of that fact.

John and I continued as before, working long hours and saving hard for our forthcoming dream holiday. As usual, I still had the best intentions to visit my mum and dad, but with a heavier workload and being exhausted most of the time, I would generally telephone them and make my excuses as to why I had not been down to see them.

"Mum, I'm totally shattered. I won't be down tonight, but I will try and get down over the weekend. Tell Dad I send my love."

On putting down the telephone receiver, I would heave a great sigh of relief at not having to go out and would then spend the rest of the evening sleeping on the sofa, only waking to the sound of John's voice telling me it was bedtime.

Waking in the mornings was also becoming a big problem for me; I just didn't have the energy to pull myself together and on most occasions would require John to constantly shout at me to get up and dressed for work. By the time I actually got myself downstairs, the tea that John had made me would be cold and there wouldn't be enough time before leaving the house to make a fresh cup, so more often than not, it would be at my work that I would have my first cup of tea to start my day.

Through the days that followed, I felt constantly tired and was now finding that when I sat down for my lunch at work, it took so much effort for me to remain awake. I remember thinking to myself, "Roseann, give yourself a shake; you're the boss and are supposed to set an example", but even those thoughts did nothing to shake off the constant feelings of fatigue that would wash over me.

By the end of a day at work, the only thing I was fit for was again a lie down on the sofa. My life was becoming one big sleep with work in between it.

John was again becoming concerned about my health, not by my ongoing problem of an inverted left nipple, but with my constant inability to stay awake; again he pressurised me into making yet another appointment to see a doctor. To be honest, I didn't know what all the fuss was about, believing that my exhaustion was down to the increase in my working hours. I had tried to explain that to John but he wouldn't listen.

"Go to the doctors, or I will lead you by the hand and take you there myself," he told me.

On entering the doctor's surgery I walked up to one of the receptionists at the main desk.

Cancer No Not Me!

"It's a young female trainee doctor that you will be seeing you today," she informed me.

"Great," I thought, "I'm never going to get out of here today," knowing from past experience that I would have to go through the rigmarole of explaining in great detail everything relating to my ongoing health problems. I felt like killing John for forcing me to go to the doctors. "I don't have time for all this palaver," I thought.

Once my name had been called and I was seated opposite the doctor, I went through the same laborious explanation about my inverted nipple, as well as the increasing feelings of tiredness I was experiencing. I also updated her on the outcome of my previous two visits to the surgery. This young inexperienced doctor informed me that she felt it best that she examine me.

The poor soul looked rather puzzled as she telephoned through to the other consultation room to request that the more experienced doctor join her, now that she had a full account of my health issues and had also now completed a full examination of my breasts.

I tried to remain calm as I sat there waiting for the other doctor to enter the room, all the while thinking of all the other things I had to do that day and of how I would have to now rush around due to being held up at the surgery. Don't get me wrong; I am a great believer in helping all new medical professionals in their quest to learn, but that day of all days was packed with things that I had to do that could not wait until my next free day off work. I also didn't know when that would be, due to the fact that I was now working any available overtime that came up, even if it happened to be on the two days that I would have normally been off in any given week.

Entering the room, I instantly recognised the male doctor as one that had been with the practice for many years. He went through the usual introductions, even though we knew each other well, before explaining that it was a standard procedure of the practice for a senior doctor to oversee new and junior doctors.

Turning to the young female doctor, he then enquired as to what my reasons were for visiting the surgery that day and her feelings on what could be the possible cause of my ongoing health problems. After explaining in great detail the problems that I had been experiencing, the young doctor then informed the other that she could find no apparent signs and symptoms during her examination of my breasts, other than my clearly noticeable inverted nipple, explaining that with so little to go on, that she was unable to make any kind of diagnosis. She then sat and waited for the other doctor to react to the way she had handled the consultation.

The more experienced doctor then went through a series of questions as to what the young doctor felt could be the root of my problems. Again, the young doctor emphasised that she could find no other signs and symptoms to assist her in a diagnosis. The more experienced doctor then turned to me to ask if there was anything further I could add as a possible explanation to my current medical problems. I told him that I had now put my nipple problem down to the weight of my breast and my tiredness to the increase in the amount of hours I was working. I then highlighted that the real reason behind my third visit to the surgery was due to my husband's concerns and insistence that I again see a doctor, because of my constant feelings of tiredness.

Cancer No Not Me!

"Do you think there is anything I should be concerned about; cancer I mean?" I asked him, thinking to myself this was the second time I'd asked that question.

After yet another examination, this time by the more experienced doctor, he also stated he could feel nothing during his examination to warrant any concern, advising me to reduce my workload and keep an eye out for any further changes in my breasts.

With that I left the surgery feeling that the whole visit had been a total waste of time, promising myself to throttle John when he came home from work for making me go to the doctor in the first place. I dismissed my problem as being nothing more than a triviality, given that all the doctors I had now seen seemed unconcerned.

I continued to sail along with my busy life, happy in the knowledge that the reasons behind my current health problems had now been pinpointed as overwork and that there was no cause for concern regarding the changes in my nipple. Any thoughts that I might have had with regard to breast cancer had also been firmly removed from my mind.

I still continued to work some extra hours to help towards our holiday fund, but on John's insistence had reduced these extra hours to no more than eight a week. To be truthful, it really didn't make a blind bit of difference to the overwhelming tiredness that I continued to experience. I now attributed the tiredness partly to getting older and not being as energetic as I used to be in my younger years.

Arranging the final details of our holiday to America was so exciting; John and I had both agreed that early November the following year would be the best time for us to go on the holiday of our dreams. Choosing that time meant that we had a full 15 months to save and plan all the things we wanted to do during our visit. The more we saved, the more excited we became. I had even started to pick up the odd top or t-shirt here and there to put by for our trip.

With regard to seeing my family, I found that it was becoming increasingly difficult. If I wasn't working, I was too tired to be bothered with general chit chat, opting to rest at every opportune moment that arose. I still telephoned my mum to check on how both she and my dad were keeping and on the odd occasion I did visit, but no sooner had I arrived at my parents' house, than I would be focusing on an acceptable time to leave. I just wanted to be in my own house, grateful at being able to curl up on the sofa and sleep.

Even when my grandchildren visited, I would find myself wishing away the hours one by one, desperately hoping that Billy our son had pre-arranged to take the girls somewhere special. Now that just was not me; I usually couldn't wait for the girls to arrive at the weekend, as I always looked forward to their visits. I enjoyed the fun that both John and I would have with the girls; we would all four of us play silly games, or paint each other's faces.

But now that had all changed. I just wasn't the fun loving gran that the girls knew anymore. Now, more often than not, I found myself becoming irritated by the little things the girls would do, whereas before I would have found their actions amusing.

As the weeks passed, I noticed that a red circle had appeared around my inverted nipple. However, as it only caused slight pain, I decided to refrain from visiting my doctor and just took some basic pain relief tablets. To be honest, I was beginning to feel that if I were to make yet another appointment to see yet another doctor about my problem, it would not have been too long before my medical records started to have "neurotic woman" recorded in them. Also, I just didn't have the time to waste, so I continued ignoring the problem.

Whilst at work one day, I began to experience a sharp pain in my left breast, which continued throughout the day. Strangely, I could neither pinpoint when it was going to happen or how long it would last. It was a piercing pain that came from deep inside my breast and straight through the nipple. These signs and symptoms actually made me sigh with relief. At last I felt I could identify what was wrong with me; an infection.

"Great," I thought, "Now I can get this problem sorted out once and for all and get on with my life; an antibiotic and I'll be fine." I didn't mind making another appointment to visit my doctor, because now I knew there was something wrong with me and I wasn't just, as I felt I had been, wasting the doctor's time.

On entering the consultation room, I was met by the more senior doctor who had seen me on my previous visit to the surgery when being seen by a junior doctor. Taking a seat, I updated him fully on the noted changes to my left breast, feeling confident that I had diagnosed my own health problem as being one of infection and actually felt quite proud of myself for doing so.

After yet another breast examination, (this was becoming a habit), my doctor informed me that with a problem such as mine, a referral to a specialist in this area would, in his opinion, be the best avenue to take. He then asked what my feelings were with regard to his suggestion.

Slightly bemused, I remember thinking to myself, "I don't think we have to go that far to treat an infection." I said that to take this avenue as a way of resolving my problem meant that time would be wasted before I would receive any treatment. I asked instead if he would prescribe me an antibiotic and some pain medication, telling him that not only would this most probably solve my health problems, but would also eliminate the need for me to visit a breast specialist. However, my opinion made no difference as my doctor informed me that he felt that he was not experienced enough in this area to be able to make a diagnosis. I did again bring up the subject of cancer, only to have our conversation redirected back to the best route being to arrange a referral to the breast clinic at our local hospital.

"This type of clinic deals with such cases sooner rather than later. You will be seen in approximately two weeks," he told me.

I knew that there was nothing else that I could do that would persuade my doctor otherwise. I left the surgery with no prescription for any of the items that I had requested, but with the knowledge that I would be attending a hospital specialist in the very near future.

On returning home from work that night John enquired about my visit.

"He's referring me to a breast clinic," I told him, rather peeved by the outcome of my visit to the surgery.

There was nothing else that I could do other than continue with the over-the-counter pain relief medication I had been taking, half hoping that in time they would solve my problem and eliminate my need to attend a clinic.

The sharp pain that would pierce through my breast was now causing me further problems by becoming more frequent, periodically disrupting my sleep. The painkillers that I had originally been taking now seemed ineffective. Into the bargain I had also now begun to snap at John for no apparent reason. I was truly becoming fed up with it all.

On one particular morning, I woke feeling rather sore and sorry for myself; the realisation that my health problems seemed to be rapidly getting worse also contributed to blackening my mood. I decided to telephone my work and take a sick day, telling myself that as it was Friday and given that I had the weekend off, I would surely feel fit enough to return to work on the Monday morning. It wasn't to be. Over the weekend things seemed to get worse; the pain and tenderness in my breast at times became unbearable and notably more regular. I did purchase a variety of pain killing drugs, but none seemed to have any effect in totally alleviating my pain. They would dull it, but even then the feelings of relief they would give me did not last for any length of time before I felt that I was back at square one.

I telephoned my work on Sunday to inform them that I would be taking a further week of sick leave. Over the next week, I experienced times when the pain in my breast was almost excruciating. My only consolation was that it seemed to go as quickly as it came, although the downside was that it was happening more frequently. I could feel myself becoming angry at the thought of my doctor leaving me in this situation for so long, especially when he could have quite easily given me an antibiotic to take away the infection that I believed was causing my problems. "I have Mastitis," I told myself. "Why my doctor cannot recognise that as the root of my problem is beyond me."

Throughout this time I chose not to go into any great depth about my health problems with my family, with the exception of John who could not help but notice the pain that I was suffering. He would constantly remark that something had to be done and I constantly reassured him, as well as myself, that it was only a matter of time until I was prescribed the appropriate medication.

Cancer No Not Me!

On Friday morning of that week, I awoke to find John getting ready for work. I felt awful and had spent most of the night in agony; whenever I had tried to turn in bed during the night, the pain in my breast would come back with a vengeance. My attitude had now changed from not wanting to visit the clinic at our local hospital, to wishing that an appointment would hurry up and arrive. I told myself, "One week down, thank God; one to go", whilst all the while thinking, "Roseann, just make it through the week and everything will be fine once an antibiotic is prescribed and starts to take effect."

No chance. Noticing the increase in pain and discomfort that I was suffering, John demanded that I return to see my general practitioner, so yet again I contacted my surgery for yet another appointment, arranging it for that day.

On arrival at the surgery, I took a seat and once again waited to see yet another doctor. It wasn't long before my name was called and I found myself again going through the now lengthy explanation as to why I had made my appointment. This doctor, like the rest before her, thoroughly examined my now very sore to the touch breast, but again I was told nothing sinister could be detected and advised I wait for the arrival of my forthcoming appointment at the hospital.

I could feel tears fill my eyes as I told her of the extreme pain in my left breast. It was apparent, however, that she did not want to override the decision of the doctor I had seen on my previous visit. She did, however, thankfully agree to write me a prescription for stronger painkillers, as well as supply me with a sick line for a further week.

Before leaving the consultation room, I did question this doctor on her thoughts of the possibilities of me having breast cancer, but really it had been a waste of time as she also was reluctant to be drawn into this form of questioning, merely opting to refer back to my forthcoming hospital appointment yet again.

I left the surgery, no further forward in my quest for antibiotics, but with both a prescription for a stronger pain killing drug and sick line for my work.

Now I know it may be hard for some people to understand why I innocently – or stupidly – plodded along unconcerned when I was in so much pain, but I had been examined so many times by different doctors at my surgery and on all occasions none of the doctors seemed to find anything to cause them concern, or highlight the possibility that I might have breast cancer. I had also been reassured frequently that no lumps had been discovered during any of my breast examinations. I was quite clearly in a lot of pain; something that I believed was not usually connected to breast cancer. Now if I had found a lump, then yes, I would have been concerned. You hear so much of, "Doctor I feel a painless lump in my breast like a small pea", as being the first sign of something suspect.

A red circle was now clearly visible around my left breast also – all the tell tale signs of an infection. Let's face it; I was only 38 years of age – too young I thought to have breast cancer.

Over the following week I felt a lot better; the pain in my breast had subsided and I felt more like my old self, something I might add that also pleased John, because not only were his fears now unfounded, he was also glad that I was not taking the face off of him whenever he opened his mouth to say something. I was well aware I had been taking all my frustrations out on him, but I just could not help myself. Well, they do say that you hurt the one you love most; poor John.

I decided to enjoy the time I had left of my sick leave now that I was pain free and happy at having some time to do all the little things at home that no one ever seems to have time to do these days because of work commitments.

On Monday morning it was back to the grind. John and I got up just as we normally did on a working day when I was on an early shift. My feelings of tiredness had diminished gradually since being prescribed a stronger painkiller. I felt satisfied that I was on the mend; even the red circle that had become a permanent fixture on my left breast did not appear as bad as it had in the past.

I wondered if this could be the end of my health problems, believing that most probably my own immune system had fought whatever infection had lurked in my breast and caused me so much grief. I watched John as he made his way to our front door to take Tess our dog out for her morning walk, whilst I went to the kitchen to put on the kettle.

Once dressed, I put on my makeup ready to face the day. I then drove John to work and, kissing him goodbye, told him I would see him later when I came to pick him up. I then continued to my own work.

John worked for our local council as a road worker and had no need for our car during the day, which worked out well because on occasions I would sometimes need the car during my working day to do application visits for those who had applied for care housing, my field of work.

On arriving at my work place, my colleagues asked how I was. I told everyone I was fine and glad to be back, before carrying on as normal. I told myself that I would get the chance later on in the day to sit down privately with my boss Maggie and update her on how I was feeling now that my health problems were almost resolved. Maggie had been a great support to me over my period of sickness; she had often telephoned to see how I was feeling and to reassure me that I didn't have to worry about work. For that, I was so very grateful.

I was surprised, however, at how concerned she still was about my breast problem and of the time it was taking for me to be seen by the breast clinic. It almost made me laugh the way she got all angry and upset; it was as if she herself was more worried than I. However, once I had reassured her that everything was fine and that I was no longer in pain, she appeared more relaxed.

I was aware at that time that I should have received word about my forthcoming hospital appointment, but to be honest, now that I was feeling better it was more the inconvenience of having to attend my hospital referral that was now praying on my mind.

As the weeks went by, I had still received no correspondence from the hospital, but this did not particularly bother me as the painkillers prescribed by the last doctor that I had seen continued to be effective; that is, with the exception of the odd shooting pain. The red circle around my left nipple continued to remain, but surely that was nothing more than my body showing it still had some infection?

A few days after returning to work, my boss Maggie enquired if I had heard anything about my forthcoming hospital appointment. On telling her that I hadn't, she instantly told me that I should wait no longer and that I should personally telephone the hospital to find out when they planned to see me. She literally went on and on about it that much, I was beginning to think that she didn't believe that I had been ill and had only fabricated my illness in order to have a few weeks off work. I know it was a terrible thought, but it did cross my mind.

Cancer No Not Me!

On Maggie's advice and her constant nagging, I eventually telephoned the hospital almost as a way of saying, "See, I told you so!" As we both sat in the office of the care house with the door shut, I dialled the hospital's number and waited for someone to answer me at the other end of the phone.

"Glasgow Royal Infirmary," I heard a female voice say. I don't know why, but I felt rather uneasy as I enquired if she could give me any information with regard to my referral. On being told to hold the line whilst she looked into the matter, I sat hand over the telephone receiver and chatted to Maggie as I waited for the telephonist to get back to me.

"Hello," said the girl. On hearing her voice, I instantly stopped talking to Maggie, re-directing my attention back to this girl on the other end of the phone. "I'm sorry," she continued, "I have no record of any referral documents in your name."

Puzzled, I asked if she would double check as I had definitely been referred some weeks prior by my doctor.

"No, I have checked; there is no record of your referral," she reiterated.

I thanked this person for their assistance and hung up the receiver.

"They have no record of any referrals in my name," I repeated back to Maggie.

"That's ridiculous! Call your doctor's surgery," she replied, pressurising me to look further into the matter.

Abruptly, I declined her advice; I was confused enough about what I had just been told without her adding to it. I told her that I would follow it up the next day. To tell you the truth, I was getting totally peed off by the whole situation.

The following morning, I got up at around 10am. I was working that day but was not due on shift until 2pm. My mind instantly started to question why the hospital had no record of me. I didn't relish the thought of yet again contacting my doctor's surgery, but I knew that I had to for my own piece of mind.

On dialling the telephone number of the surgery, I felt nervous, imagining that on hearing that it was me on the other end of the telephone, the receptionist would instantly think to herself, "Oh, it's her again". I know that may sound silly, but given that I wasn't usually someone to regularly visit their doctor, these thoughts did go through my mind. Funny how your mind can play tricks on you like that; it wasn't as if I was a person who had not been familiar with talking to doctors and their receptionists. I worked in the care sector and spoke with doctors and their colleagues on a daily basis, but then again it had never been about me.

When the receptionist answered, I quickly babbled out why I was telephoning. It was almost as if I felt the quicker I got the words out, the quicker I would have an answer and the better I would then feel, if that makes any sense. I was shocked to discover, however, that my hospital referral had only been requested a few days earlier. This meant that all the time that I had been painstakingly waiting for my appointment to arrive by post, when I had been feeling at my worst, they hadn't even contacted the hospital. Talk about being angry; I was fuming!

In order to make sense of it all, I told myself that doctors have so much to deal with in one day that it must be easy for something to slip their mind.

What I will say is that this experience has taught me never to hesitate in contacting doctors, clinics and other medical professionals in relation to my own health or that of a family member. This could have been a situation where my referral could have so easily been a matter of urgency.

Ironically, the following day I received a letter informing me that an appointment had been made for me to attend the breast clinic at the hospital the forthcoming week.

Chapter Two

Realising the Truth

My eldest sister Issy lived across the road from me and after telling her of the trouble I had been having with my health, as well as informing her that I was to attend a clinic at our local hospital, she promptly said she would go with me. I knew what she would automatically be thinking; cancer! Therefore, I reassured her that I had no lumps in my breasts and told her how all the doctors I had seen had eliminated any possibility of breast cancer. To be honest, I really felt there was no need for her to come with me. I had already told John that I didn't need him to be there as I now felt much better and was only really going to be prescribed an antibiotic to clear up any infection that may have still been present in my breast. I repeated this to my sister, hoping I could persuade her against coming with me to my appointment, but you know what sisters are like; she told me we could make a day of it and have lunch in town after my appointment. I knew this was only her way of making sure I could not decline her offer, so in the end I accepted and waited for the day of my appointment to arrive.

Back at work, I told Maggie of how I had now received the details of when I should attend the clinic, informing her I would arrange to take annual leave for that day. She would not hear of it, telling me that I would take the day as sick leave, which made me feel rather odd given that there was not much wrong with me.

I have always been one of those people who feel guilty when taking time off work and that day was no different, but with

Cancer No Not Me!

Maggie's authorisation, I was actually quite pleased at knowing that I had the whole day to spend in town after the clinic. It was great; almost like having a free day off work for nothing.

The following week sailed along as usual. John and I worked hard and, like most days, returned home and both happily nodded off after our supper. On the odd occasion I felt tired, but in no way was it anything like the exhaustion I had experienced in the past, which pleased me. I still experienced pain in my left breast, but the painkillers seemed to be keeping the pain at a tolerable level.

Work, plus everything else that was going on in life, never really gave me much time to dwell on my health problems, putting them most of the time to the back of my mind.

It's strange, but I couldn't really take my health problems seriously. Whether or not I was unconsciously refusing to face my situation, I truthfully do not know. Maybe as individuals we have an automatic escape valve built deep inside us that enables us to mask our fears when we are unable to face them. Who knows?

Finally, the day of my appointment arrived; 17th November 1999. I had slept well the night before and was glad of the extra time I had managed to get in bed, feeling good at not having to work that day. John and I had discussed my hospital appointment the previous night and I had reassured him once again that I did not need him to come with me. So as I lay in my bed that morning, John kissed me goodbye on his way to work and wished me luck. He then left the house as I stayed in bed promising myself another hour, enjoying the fact that I had a day to do what I wanted after I had got this stupid hospital appointment out of the way.

I got up around 8am, showered and walked over to my sister's house. My appointment was for around 10.30am and we had both decided go to the hospital by bus rather than drive; that way we could spend the day window shopping without having to worry about parking, plus we could enjoy a nice pub lunch and most probably an alcoholic beverage before returning home.

So, all dressed up, off we went to start our day. Funny how you have to always make sure you have clean underwear on when going to see a doctor!

Issy and I arrived early at the hospital, so we decided to go to the canteen for some breakfast. Whilst in there, we noticed an attractive girl sitting by herself. I remember commenting on her figure and appearance, half wishing I too had a figure like hers. We went to the breakfast bar to choose what we wanted to eat and then sat down and began to plan our shopping trip. I thought no more about the girl.

Arriving at the clinic, I presented my appointment card to the girl at the reception desk of clinic one, then both Issy and I took a seat in the waiting area. I remember looking up at the sign that said, "Oncology". Now anyone that did not work within the care profession would most probably not have given that sign a second thought, but I felt a strange feeling of uneasiness. To me, oncology and cancer were one and the same thing. Trying to dismiss the thoughts of fear that were beginning to enter my head – "Cancer! Cancer! Cancer!" – I found my attention wandering back to the previous week.

On hearing that I had to attend a breast clinic, one of my fellow colleagues at work informed me that she had once been sent to one for investigation of a lump that had appeared in her breast. She explained to me that she had been given what was known as a needle test. She then proceeded to tell me exactly what the test entailed, choosing

Cancer No Not Me!

to include all the gory details in her explanation. "Roseann, it was agony; they had to hold me down, as I screamed at the top of my voice," she said.

To be honest, with no signs of a lump in my breast, I had been unconcerned about her comments at that time, but now I had begun to reflect on what she had told me.

"Roseann Gallagher!"

I was jolted from my thoughts by my name being called. On rising from my seat, I handed my sister my coat and handbag and walked in the direction of this woman calling my name. Introducing herself as Jean, she explained that she was a breast nurse based at the clinic. She then proceeded to direct me to a consultation room.

As I entered the room, I could plainly see an examination table at one side of the room and a desk with some chairs opposite. Again, the nurse spoke, this time to ask that I remove all my clothing from the upper half of my body and put on an examination gown stating, "The doctor will be in to see you shortly." She then left the room. I did as I was instructed, then popped my bottom onto the edge of the examination table, not really knowing what to do as I waited.

I remember thinking that maybe I should have brought Issy into the examination room with me, but then again I didn't know if that would have been allowed. It's funny when in a situation like this how very vulnerable you feel, almost like being a child again.

The door of the consultation room opened and in walked the nurse and another female; the girl we had seen in the canteen! The woman introduced herself as Alison Lanagan, then told me that she was the consultant that would be dealing with my case. She obviously did not recognise me from earlier that morning in the same way that both my sister and I had noticed her. This woman must have been in her mid-twenties and had an air about her that instantly made you feel at ease. Standing beside me, she asked what problems I had been experiencing with regard to my breasts and general health, adding that she also wished me to inform her of any medication I might have been taking.

I updated her on all the events that had happened since the start of dilemma and proceeded to inform her of my thoughts on the whole issue.

"I think I have developed an infection in my left breast," I told her. "Possibly Mastitis," I continued.

The silence seemed to last forever before finally she spoke.

"Would you mind if I examined your breasts, Mrs. Gallagher?" she asked me.

On telling her I had no objection to an examination, she then asked that I sit at the edge of the examination table and remove my gown. I was asked to relax my arm in hers as she proceeded to examine first my left breast and then the right, all the while saying nothing. I watched her face hoping to see a smile, but it remained expressionless.

I began to feel myself becoming tense at the time it was taking for the doctor to complete a rather simple examination, unsure as to why I required such an in-depth check.

"Is there any history of breast cancer in your family?" she enquired.

Now that certainly did make me feel anxious and instantly made me take more notice of what the doctor said and the way in which she continued to re-examine each of my breasts. Frightening thoughts began running through my head. Throughout the consultation, the breast care nurse remained in the room.

Cancer No Not Me!

So there I was, sitting at the edge of an examination table expecting a quick check-up, followed by a prognosis of inflammation of the breast. Wrong! After finishing her examination and whilst I was still perched at the end of the examination table, this woman informed me that during her examination she had detected a lump in my left breast. I couldn't believe my ears; surely she must be mistaken? After all, I had been to four other doctors within such a short period of time and none of them had felt anything.

She continued by then informing me that I would require further tests in order to enable her to fully diagnose what was wrong with me, startling me more by telling me that she wanted me to have the tests completed after she had finished her consultation with me. Firstly, I was to have what was known as a mammogram, a standard test given to women to detect any signs of lumps in the breast. Secondly, I was to have a needle test, the same test that my friend Noreen had explained to me in great depth. "Thanks Noreen", I remember thinking.

My mind by this time was racing at a hundred miles an hour; mammogram/needle test. I felt totally helpless at that moment and to be honest was becoming more anxious by the minute. All the while the breast nurse remained by my side, almost like a crutch at the ready just in case I should crumble. My mind raced to thoughts of Issy, who was still sitting in the waiting area unaware of what was going on.

The consultant took a seat at her desk and began to write, whilst I slowly got dressed. Once fully clothed, I then took the seat opposite the doctor. I felt numb whilst the appropriate documentation was being completed for the tests that I now required. Handing the completed paperwork to me, the doctor jolted me from an almost hypnotic state of panic that had now begun to rise within me.

After taking the relevant documents from her hand, I was then guided by the breast care nurse out of the examination room and given directions to the x-ray department, a totally different direction I might add from the waiting area where I had left my sister. I walked to the x-ray department in a complete daze and once there tried to logically analyse everything the doctor had said to me.

It's strange how many feelings and emotions can go through someone's mind simultaneously. I experienced denial, fear, helplessness, panic and terror. I had feelings of wanting to run away, but where would I go? I was slowly falling apart at the seams. My ability to cope seemed to be draining from my body, but at the same time I also knew I had to be strong, if not for myself, then for my sister.

Some of you reading this book will know and understand these feelings well and most probably relate to what I am trying to say. I know that people feel terrible emotional turmoil when being told of a loved one's diagnosis of cancer, but to possibly be a victim of this terrible disease myself was one of the most awful feelings that anyone can experience.

Tears started to trickle down my face uncontrollably as I again thought of my sister; an overwhelming need to have her by my side engulfed me. Thoughts of, "What do I say?" and "How do I say it?" ran through my mind, which only added to my distress. My thoughts continued to race in a spiral decent: "Issy, they've found a lump. I'm sure they think it's cancer. I'm frightened to death; please take these awful feelings away and make everything alright again." I felt so helpless.

Rising to my feet, I sped in the direction of the breast clinic waiting area, informing the receptionist of the x-ray department whilst in motion that I would not be long. I felt almost like a doll that had been wound up from behind, as I tried so hard to control my emotions. The walk from the x-ray department to the clinic was only a few yards, but believe me, it felt like a mile.

Issy was glancing through a magazine as I approached her. She looked surprised to see me coming towards her from a totally different direction from which I had originally gone. I gestured to her to follow me. With a puzzled expression she stood up and began to walk beside me as I made my way back to the x-ray department.

It's strange how you try to remain calm and brave. When I reflect on that moment, something that will live with me for the rest of my life, I now realise that we all must have this inbred need to protect our own. It was a curious feeling, in that although this terrible experience was happening to me, my natural instinct was to appear strong and protect my sister; it was almost like having an invisible inner strength that we do not even realise exists until we have to extract from it. The last thing I wanted was for Issy to experience the emotional turmoil that I was already enduring.

My mind drifted back to all the people sitting in the clinic waiting area. I could now empathise with them and understand their fears and anxieties.

As we walked in the direction of the x-ray department, I began to tell my sister briefly what had gone on during my consultation.

"The doctor said that she could feel a lump in my breast."

There, I got it out without crying.

"I have to have further tests to detect whether or not I have cancer," I continued.

It was becoming increasingly difficult to speak, as if my throat was slowly closing. I was silenced by the tears that had begun to fill my eyes and as we walked arm in arm, no more words were needed.

We sat in the x-ray department waiting area. Breaking the silence, I told my sister how frightened I now felt.

"Everything will be fine," she reassuringly told me, but I could see by her expression that she was now having problems trying to digest the information I had just given her. I watched her as she tried to remain calm, but behind her expression I could clearly see she was trying her best to be strong for me.

When you are at your most frightened, you seem to totally home in on your loved ones, hoping to see a different expression or hear different words from the ones you yourself would convey if in their situation. Then, of course, when you see them trying so very hard to hide their emotions and fears by expressing a positive attitude to the situation you are in, you worry even more because not only do you think your world is falling apart, they think it is too, which in turn only adds to your helplessness!

Again, my name was called, this time by a radiographer of the x-ray department and again I followed as instructed. On entering the mammogram room, I was asked to strip to the waist then walk towards and stand directly facing a monstrous machine in the centre of the room that I could only presume would be taking the x-rays of my breasts.

Being instructed by the Radiographer, I was told to wrap my arms around the machine as far as they would stretch. At the same time, the radiographer positioned my left breast on a small cold metal shelf-like platform. My breast was then firmly held in place between two metal plates and x-rayed. The whole procedure was once again repeated, but this time with my right breast. I now scanned the radiographer's facial expression, but was unable to extract anything from it.

Once my x-rays were completed, I was instructed to get dressed and then told to return to the waiting area of the x-ray department where the radiographer would bring me the developed x-rays of my breasts for me to take back to the clinic, to be studied by Alison Lanagan. On receipt of my x-rays, both Issy and I walked back to the clinic where my whole nightmare had begun.

The receptionist told me to take a seat whilst she informed the staff at the clinic. In no time at all, Jean – the breast care nurse – returned to the waiting area and asked me to join her as Issy remained behind. I was then taken to yet another room, this time to have the dreaded needle test that my friend had so candidly described to me. As I walked towards the examination bed, the nurse remained by my side. She again reminded me that her name was Jean and reassured me that the test was not that bad and would be over rather quickly. A different female doctor from the one that I had seen earlier had already prepared the things she would need in order to obtain the required samples.

Again, I was required to undress the upper half of my body and put on yet another hospital gown. I then made my way as instructed to the examination couch, then sat half upright with my gown opened at the front. The doctor did give me her name, but it didn't register in my head; I was too anxious about what was going on around me.

I suppose as I think back, the only consolation for me at that time was that Jean was at my side. Terrified, I had asked her if she would hold my hand whilst I was having the procedure done; something I did not have to request twice, because within an instant her hand was in mine. Her actions I will never forget, as at that moment I desperately needed someone. As instructed by the doctor, who was also at my side, I nervously lay back on the bed and tried to relax, but it was impossible.

Slowly, the doctor explained the test to me; a small needle would be inserted into the area of my left breast that had been identified as having the lump. A very small section – about the size of a pinhead – would be removed in order to test for cancerous cells. I was told that two samples would be required; again it was reinforced to me that the whole procedure would be over in a matter of minutes.

Nervously, I asked the doctor to inform me when she was about to take her sample; I needed time to prepare myself. So with Jean's hand in mine, I was ready for the doctor to begin.

Now I know it could be beneficial to those of you who may one day, like I, have to go through this procedure, to gain an insight into what this test entails. Therefore, to put you in the picture and also help blow away any myths or horror stories like the one I was told, here is a true account of what happens.

Firstly, the needle that is used for this procedure is very small – approximately an inch if my memory serves me well. Secondly, the test is as both the nurse and doctor explained, over as quickly as it began and, thirdly, the test in my opinion was not as my friend had described; "that bad that you have to be held down" or "that painful that it makes you scream in pain". You do feel a rather sharp nip, almost like getting an injection and then it's over. The taking of the second sample is not as bad as the first, because then you know exactly what to expect. I do have to say there was some pain, but please let me reassure you that it was not as my friend had described. It was nothing that even the most squeamish of individuals could not tolerate.

When I think back in more depth to that particular test, I think the reason why we experience some of the pain we do is mainly down to our instinct to fear the unknown; this inevitably causes us to tense up inside and that in turn elicits feelings of panic that makes us more sensitive to pain. I do believe that never a truer statement has been made than that of: "If you just relax, it will make it easier for you."

This is something that I now try my utmost to do when faced with the prospect of any form of test or procedure. Believe me, it works! Clear your mind of everything other than your breathing; focus on the in and out motion of your breathing. As you take that big breath in, think of all the little air sacks in your lungs that swell up, happy at receiving the thing that keeps them alive and as you release that breath, visualise in your mind's eye how by doing this simple action you rid your body of all its impurities. Thus, by focusing all your energy and thoughts on only your breathing, you also leave little or no space in your mind to host anxious thoughts.

After the completion of my needle tests, I was then escorted by Jean back to the waiting area and informed that I would be called again as soon as my samples had been analysed.

On returning to the waiting area, I joined Issy who had anxiously been waiting for my return. I told her the details of the tests and how it was only a matter of waiting until the results were concluded.

"They said in about 10 minutes," I explained to her anxiously.

We then just sat there in silence; there was nothing else we could do other than wait.

Out of the blue, our silence was broken.

"Have you been examined yet?" were the words from another female waiting to be seen. At first, I instinctively thought "How dare this woman have the cheek to ask about my business?" but as I looked at her closely, I could see the fear in her eyes, realising that she had spoken only through concern. "If only she knew," I remember thinking to myself.

I smiled at her sympathetically as I informed her that, yes, I had already been seen by the doctor and was now waiting for the results of the tests, reassuring her that both the mammogram x-ray and the needle test had not been that bad, hoping that would be the end of the conversation.

Normally, I was the type of person that could usually talk for Britain, but not on that day; I just wasn't in the mood. "No such luck," I thought, as the woman then began to tell both my sister and I in great detail the reason for her visit. She told of how she had bumped her breast, how a lump had appeared and how her doctor had referred her to the clinic more as a precaution, rather than of worry that there could be something sinister. The more she talked, the more terrified she appeared. I explained, without going into any great detail, almost as a way of trying to calm this poor woman, that the staff were extremely supportive and if she did require the tests that I had just had then she needn't worry.

It's curious how some things can avert us from our own worries. There I was with thoughts running wild in my head about the outcome of my test results, yet I was actually appearing calm as a cucumber reassuring this lady.

"Roseann Gallagher," called Jean from the clinic area.

I quickly rose to my feet, again leaving my sister to sit in the waiting area. As I began to walk towards Jean, I continually repeated in my head, "It's not cancer, it's not cancer."

I looked at Jean's face in the hope of being able to determine my results from the expression on her face, but she gave nothing away. However, I did feel slightly relieved that she didn't have one of those sad, sympathetic looks. If she had, then I would have been worried. I quickened my step, keen to put the whole sorry episode behind me. However, as I approached the nurse she continued to look in my direction, but I quickly realised not at me, but beyond me. As I turned to see what had attracted her attention, I then realised that it was Issy. She was looking at Issy. I started to feel uneasy.

"Is that your sister?" she asked.

On hearing those words, the hair on the back of my neck stood up and once again I was in a situation where fear overwhelmed me. Earlier during my consultation, the doctor had enquired if I was on any medication, to which I replied that I was and that I had brought it with me. When I had been informed that I required further tests, I had asked Jean if she would give my medication to my sister as it would save me from having to carry it around in my hand. I had even jokingly told Jean, "You can't miss her; my mum had five girls and we all look alike." So when Jean had then enquired if Issy was indeed my sister, she already knew the answer to her own question, because she had exchanged words earlier with her when handing her my medication.

I was now becoming seriously worried, even more so when asked if I would like my sister to join us. Well on hearing that, I was practically rooted to the spot as I continually tried to analyse why the nurse was keen for Issy to join us. I tried to make sense of it all, but the only conclusion I was coming up with was the last thing I wanted to hear. I would never have believed that so many thought processes could go through one's head in such a short space of time.

I looked in the direction of my sister and gestured with my hand for her to join us. Thoughts of "I have to be brave, I have to be brave," were running through my head, whilst at the same time I had this terrible fear of knowing that something was seriously wrong.

Although the consultation room was only a few feet away, the walk seemed to take forever; it was as if I were going in slow motion. However, my heart and mind were racing so very, very fast. "Cancer! Cancer! Cancer! I've got it. Why else would this nurse be suggesting that I ask my sister to join me to hear my results? She hadn't suggested Issy accompany me whilst I went through the tests I required," I thought.

As we entered the consultation room, my instinct told me that the news was not going to be good. The doctor that had been dealing with my case was sitting at her desk. Jean gestured to us to take a seat, whilst she moved in the direction of the doctor and stood behind her.

"I take it that it's bad news then," I heard myself say to the doctor.

God only knows where those words came from; it was not exactly the most appropriate statement to make, but I can only put it down to nerves. Or maybe it was because I truly hoped the answer to my question would be, "No, not at all Mrs. Gallagher; your test results are clear."

As the doctor lifted her head to look at me, she began to speak.

"I am sorry Mrs. Gallagher, the news is not good."

In making that statement, the doctor was only confirming what I had now begun to suspected; CANCER. As my sister and I sat in silence, waiting to hang onto every word that would now come from this woman's lips, I could feel the tension heighten. The doctor went on to inform me that the results of my tests had confirmed that I did have cancer. I was numb. The only things that registered in my brain now were thoughts of "I'm dying," and "I'm not ready to die. I have so many things to do; my family needs me." It was almost as if I was telepathically telling God that the things I had to deal with in life far outweighed the possibility of – and reasons for – my death.

I do not know whether this was deliberate or not, but the way the chairs had been positioned in the consultation room were in such a way that I directly faced the consultant, Alison Lanagan. However, the seat offered to my sister was positioned behind and slightly to the side of me. This meant that with the chairs being positioned in this manner, neither my sister nor I could see each other face to face, unless I physically turned around to Issy, or she bent forward to look at me. Whether or not intentional by the clinic staff, this turned out to be something for which I was truly grateful. I knew that if I had physically looked directly at Issy as the consultant spoke, I would have most definitely gone to pieces. Thus, the arrangement of seating gave me a few moments in which to try to compose myself before inevitably turning around to face her.

I clearly remember at that point trying to hide my expression of sheer disbelief. However, something that I could not hide were the floods of tears that had begun to run down my face.

When I did eventually speak, the only words I could say were, "Issy, you'd better not cry." I needed to be brave for my sister, strange as it may seem; you never want to see your own suffer. God only knows what was running through my sister's mind; from that day to this, I have never asked her. Anyway, a fruitless statement it was indeed, because by this time our tears had minds of their own and continued running down both our faces, no matter how hard we both tried to stop them.

My thoughts turned to John and how we had kissed each other goodbye that morning, oblivious to the terrible news that lay ahead of us. How I wished at that moment he was by my side.

I turned my attention back to the consultant, who had been speaking continually throughout my rapid thought processes. I could hear her inform me that I would require surgery and possibly radiotherapy treatment. Again, my thoughts ran riot and I found myself thinking back to the doctors that I had seen at the Health Centre as well as the wasted weeks of waiting that I had endured. I stopped the consultant in mid-conversation.

"If my lump had been detected earlier i.e. by the doctors at my health centre, would my prognosis have had a better outcome?" I asked.

Her answer to my question was an emphatic "No", explaining that I could have had cancer from anywhere between seven months to two years. I was horrified. She then resumed her discussion with me about the surgery and treatment that lay ahead. Again, her words were interrupted, but this time by a gentleman who had just entered the room. Introducing himself as Professor Cooke, he informed me that he was the head of the department for Breast Cancer Care. "I must be bad," I remember thinking to myself. Taking my hand for a moment, he stated that he was very sorry to hear of the news that I had just received. He then informed me that Alison Lanagan had updated him fully on the results that I had just received. He said that my ability to take in all the information would most probably be affected due to the shock of hearing my results. How right he was.

My thoughts were continuing to run at a thousand miles an hour by this point. The conversation then turned to an explanation of the options that were open to me with regards to my prognosis. "Oh, God, here it comes," I thought. Firstly, I was informed that Alison would be completing any surgery that I required. I felt momentary relief at hearing that, as strangely I had begun to warm to this person and felt as confident as I could, given the circumstances.

Alison Lanagan then took up the conversation by explaining that both she and Professor Cooke felt that there were two possible avenues to take with regard to my treatment. The first option entailed a complete Lumpectomy – the removal of my tumour – and also the removal of all lymph nodes under my left armpit. The other option would be a mastectomy – the removal of my full breast – and again complete removal of lymph nodes.

The Professor jotted a few diagrams down showing both procedures, all the while assuring me as he did so that there were many treatments for my condition and that the progress in the treatment of breast cancer had developed dramatically over the last ten years. His words gave me a momentary feeling of hope. He then rose to his feet and politely excused himself before leaving the room.

I was informed that I would be required to return to the hospital the following day for more in depth biopsies. Everything was now beginning to becoming so real. Dates were now also mentioned for my forthcoming surgery. By this time, I was finding it increasingly difficult to keep up with the conversation, although I did hear the end of the month being mentioned.

Suddenly, an image of my son Billy flashed through my mind. America! That's where he was visiting a friend. I couldn't go through an operation without seeing my son. What if I died? The need to see him overwhelmed me.

I turned to Alison and started to speak. In sheer panic, I explained about my son being overseas and my need to see him before I could even contemplate having surgery. She informed me that the decision was mine. Mine? I didn't know if I was coming or going and the decision was mine. I felt helpless.

After a silence that seemed to go on forever, Alison Lanagan then asked when my son was due to return home. On informing her the beginning of December, she then again looked at her diary and after some thought informed me that putting my surgery back a further week would not change the situation that I was in. Therefore, given the circumstances, my first surgery date originally suggested was cancelled and another one was arranged; 3 December 1999. She even arranged for me not to be admitted to hospital until the morning of my operation to allow me more time to spend with my son prior to my surgery.

"Roseann," Alison told me, "as long as you come into the ward a few days before your surgery for blood tests and, given that all is well – oh, and if you also promise not to eat after midnight of that evening – then I will arrange for you to be admitted at 8am on the day of your surgery."

I was so truly grateful for her compassion.

The conversation then returned to the subject of the more in-depth biopsies that I was to have the following day. I was informed that I should attend clinic four on my arrival at the hospital, a thought that I did not relish. Thoughts of the lady we had spoken to earlier in the waiting area of the clinic flashed through my mind. I imagined what her expression would have been at seeing the state I was in. I knew that if I were to come face to face with her, she would have anxiously enquired as to how I had got on. There was no way I could have faced seeing this woman again. I suddenly froze and on seeing me do so, Jean asked me what was wrong. On telling her my feelings on having to pass this woman in the waiting area, she instantly ushered us out of the clinic via another exit, giving us both the privacy we so desperately needed.

Once outside, I found myself looking at everyone going busily about their own business, trying to imagine how anyone of them would have felt, or in what way they would have reacted to receiving the news that I had just been told. It's strange, but I then began to wonder what tragic things, if any, were going on in their individual lives and, if none, how lucky they were. It's rather strange how bad news makes one look at everything in a different light. You see, on thinking back, I know that if I had received the results that I had expected, I would have most probably left that hospital that day giving none of those people a second thought. Walking along the road, all I could think of was that I was going to die, together with thoughts of everything that I had done in my life and thoughts of my family.

It's funny how we, as humans, constantly go through life putting off all the things we dream of doing, assuming that there will always be a "tomorrow". We always seem to have something more important to do, or some other avenue for our money to go down. It's not until life slaps you hard on the face that you realise just how short life actually is and how silly you have been not to have fulfilled your dreams.

Still holding tightly onto my sister's arm, we walked in the direction of town.

"Issy, do you think I am going to die?" I asked my sister.

I could not help myself. I knew that her answer would be "No", even if she had thought otherwise, but I felt I needed to hear my sister tell me that everything would be alright. She did reply as I expected and as she did tears once again began to slowly run down my face as we continued walking.

Chapter Three

A Maze of Muddle

The urge to continue our day as planned overwhelmed me; it was almost as if this was a way of escape for me. By continuing the day as it had originally been arranged felt almost like a way of eluding the reality of all that had happened, something I am sure Issy found hard to understand. However, those thoughts did not last long and before I knew it I was telling my sister that I no longer wanted to continue our shopping trip, putting it on the back burner in favour of heading straight to the nearest pub for a few stiff drinks.

It's hard to explain, but my feeling of wanting to run away had now become even stronger, almost to a state of sheer panic. It felt like I was stuck in a maze not knowing which way I should turn to enable me to find release from my tormentor.

On entering the first pub that came our way, Issy went to the bar whilst I searched for a secluded corner away from prying eyes. The last thing I wanted was other people's stares transfixed on both of us, wondering what was wrong, something that would have been evident given that my face was still very red and puffy from my ocean of tears.

Shortly joined again by Issy, I could see she had two rather large drinks in hand.

"I got us both a double," she told me, as she took the seat next to mine.

On handing me one of the glasses, we both instantly took a large gulp almost in the hope that surely this would help to ease our pain, but alas, no such luck. Even the alcohol was hard to swallow and I found myself forcing it down my throat rather than enjoying it.

My thoughts again wandered as I found myself pondering the heartbreak that lay ahead. Thinking of my son in America, I wondered how the hell I was going to tell him I had cancer. I shared these thoughts with my sister. We talked about a member of the family telephoning Billy in America to break the news, but I didn't want that; there was no way that I could bear to think of my son having to travel home from such a faraway place with so many hours to mull over this terrible turmoil. I then knew for sure that I would insist that no one utter a word to Billy with regard to my illness; that is, until John told him on his return home. I felt so much better after making that decision. I made my sister promise me that she would ensure that no one in our family would contact Billy behind my back to tell him. Issy seemed to understand as she told me how she would feel exactly the same way in my situation.

Finishing the drinks that were in front of us, I rose to my feet to go to the bar. I just needed to be doing something; it was as if I were a hamster in a wheel running and running and getting nowhere. I just didn't know what to do.

Within moments of returning from the bar with two more drinks in my hand, however, I knew I no longer wanted to be there. I just wanted to go home where I felt safe. On expressing this to Issy, we both picked up our jackets and bags, then made our way out of the pub. Walking into the street, I could feel the freshness of the air instantly hit my face. Taking a deep breath, I found it hard to accept that now I could so easily be sentenced to having only a few more of these experiences.

My thoughts turned to Maggie. She would be sitting at work wondering how I had got on.

"Issy, I want to telephone my work from one of those payphones," I told my sister, pointing to the telephone booths on the opposite side of the road.

It was as if I so desperately needed to put everything in order, almost as if I now felt time was of the essence. I also knew that by speaking to Maggie on a public telephone I would have control of when the conversation would end, enabling me only to convey a short message of how I was now going on long term sick leave and the reason why. I felt physically sick as I dialled the number, knowing that from then on there was no turning back. There would be no statements of, "Would you believe it? They made a mistake; I don't have cancer." Realisation of my situation was well and truly sinking in.

Jolted back to reality by Maggie's voice on the other end of the telephone, I swallowed hard to remove an imaginary lump that had suddenly formed in my throat. Quickly and without feeling, I managed to blurt out my diagnosis of breast cancer. I now realise she suspected the worst all along. My ability to function was fast deteriorating as I mixed up my words and repeated myself, but that did not matter, because the outcome was the same; off work due to cancer.

On exiting the phone box, I saw a taxi and quick as a flash I put my hand up to halt it. Poor Issy; I think she was totally confused by my actions, never knowing what to expect from one minute to the next. How she coped with being in that situation of chaos I will never know. I just felt I didn't know where to turn, or what to do next and when I did decide to do something, like continue my shopping trip, for example, I immediately lost all interest.

The journey in the taxi seemed endless. As I stared out of the window watching everyone go by, I could recall experiencing the feeling of not understanding how these people could continue regardless, whilst I had this terrible burden to carry. The only other time I have ever experienced these feelings was whilst sitting in a car on my way to the funeral of a close member of my family.

I was soon at it again.

"Issy, we need to stop and pick up some alcohol; I have none in the house", I told her, almost in a panic.

I needed a few stiff drinks to see me through the next few hours whilst I waited for John to return home from work. I was also pinning my hopes on the alcohol helping me blot out my feelings of despair, whether I was in the mood for it or not.

I remember handing my sister my purse, not caring how much she spent or on what, whilst I waited in the taxi. On her return, we continued our journey back to my house. Getting out of the taxi, I remember looking up to meet the driver's eyes, thinking to myself, "He must be disgusted at these two woman buying alcohol at that time of the day."

Once in the safe enclosure of my home and with a drink in hand, I tried to think about the situation rationally, but I couldn't, no matter how hard I tried. Before long, I found myself in floods of tears and babbling to my sister that all that lay in front of me now was impending death, whilst Issy tried her best to reassure me that everything would be alright and that I wasn't going to die.

Between our tears we spoke of how best to break the news of my cancer to the rest of the family. I had already decided that my son would be told on his return home from America, but what about John? How was I going to tell him the news and what of poor mum and dad? I recalled how my mum would often comment on how no parent should have to suffer living with the death of a child; she would often make that statement when reading articles or hearing news of some poor woman in that situation, stating "I could never live with that happening to me." Little did she know that one of her worst nightmares might just unfold in front of her and the thought of telling her broke my heart.

My sisters would also have to be told, as would my granddaughters and even my nieces and nephews. Things were becoming more and more complicated by the minute; it was all just getting to much to bear.

My mother once again came into my thoughts. I remember thinking about how, as we get older, we seem to reverse roles with our parents; we become the protectors and our parents become the ones who need looking after. With this in mind, I knew in my heart I could not tell my mother my awful news, not until she had my dad by her side. However, my mother later told me that by withholding the news from her until my father had returned home from work, I had not only added to her worry, but I contributed to making my mother's day almost as awful as my own.

Issy broke my thoughts.

"Roseann, I'm just going over to my house to pick up Tara as she has been in the house all day alone."

Tara was my sister's boxer dog.

"I will take Tess with me; they both need a walk," she told me.

"Thank you," I thought to myself, as there was no way that I wanted to leave my house. I did not relish the thought of bumping into one of my neighbours.

I felt so alone when my sister left the house and my thoughts ran through the possible outcome of my situation.

Maybe if they took the lump out, that would be the end of it. I then thought to myself that cancer spreads like wildfire and that once you've got it, very few people escape it. Then I tried to reassure myself that that wasn't true. No matter how hard I tried, I couldn't prevent my thoughts from returning to the possibility of my death. Being alone was almost unbearable and I found myself looking at the clock and wishing that Issy was back. She seemed to be taking forever; or it just felt like that to me.

The front door of my house opened and in Issy walked followed by two excited dogs. How glad I was to see them return. Talk about unconditional love; it just poured from our pets.

"What took you so long?" I asked my sister, almost in a state of panic at having been left with only my thoughts to keep me company.

"I met one of our neighbours," she explained.

The thought horrified me. What came next was even worse.

"I told her about you being diagnosed with cancer," she told me.

I could have killed her, especially when John and other members of my own family had not been told. Can you imagine John returning home from work only to be approached by a neighbour expressing condolences at hearing I had cancer? That was the thought now going through my head and it terrified me. In Issy's defence though, I can understand the turmoil and devastation she must have been feeling and her need to share with someone.

I don't know to this day what possessed me not to contact John at his work that day, a decision I now truly regret. Looking back on the situation, I knew that it should have been John who was sitting there with me that day and not my sister, but it wasn't. He should have been the one doing all the tasks that I was now asking my sister to do, like telephoning other family members to inform them of my illness. Why I had asked my sister to do this is beyond me. I can only assume that I believed I was protecting John from some of our heartache. However, on reflection I now feel that my actions had the opposite effect, because I robbed John of his role as a loving husband as well as my next of kin. I realise now that I took that responsibility from under his feet. Given the opportunity to take control of the situation most likely would have also helped him to cope better with his own emotions. I can see and understand that now. I am truly sorry John.

Sitting opposite my sister in the lounge of my house, we talked about everything and nothing, trying to be jovial for each other, but anything we tried to make sound funny just seemed to fall flat and dwindle into a terrible silence. We were both physically and mentally exhausted.

I visualised John entering the house, but no matter how hard I tried, I was unable to contemplate what would happen next.

"Issy, how am I going to tell John?" I heard myself say, as alcohol began to take control of me.

On suggesting that she tell John for me, I literally jumped down her throat.

"No! I will tell him myself," I told her.

This was something that I had to do on my own, something very personal that could not just be said as it had been to the family members to whom Issy had spoken earlier on the phone. This was solely between John and me.

Everything was beginning to become all too much for me and I felt physically sick every time I thought of John walking through the door. Yes, I desperately wanted him home and by my side, but at the same time, by not having him at home, I felt as if I was protecting him from the nightmare.

Between the alcohol that I had been swallowing at an alarming rate and further thoughts of the reality of my situation, I just felt I could take no more. Uncontrollable tears ran down my face once again and I began to cry hysterically. Getting to her feet, my sister walked over to where I was sitting, sat beside me hugged me closely as she joined in my despair.

Time went so slowly. At around 3.40pm, the front door of my house opened and in walked my young niece, Issy's daughter. She had returned from school and on finding her mother not at home, knew that she would either be with me, or else I would have known where to get her. Oblivious to what had happened that day, we sat her down and tried to calmly tell her about my cancer diagnosis. At seeing how upset I was, my niece calmly informed me that with regard to my forthcoming surgery for breast cancer, it was only a boob and who cared as long as I was still alive. "The truth from mouths of babes does come," I remember thinking, as all three of us burst into laughter. Amazing how children look at things from a totally different angle to we adults.

By 4pm I felt physically sick knowing that John would be home approximately 15 minutes later. I paced the floor. I had hoped the alcohol I had been drinking all afternoon would have dulled the pain and made it easier for me to cope. How wrong I was. If anything, it had only added to my fears and emotions as I anxiously waited for John. Walking towards the window, I caught sight of our car entering the drive. John was home.

I will never forget the expression on his face as he entered the house, not amused at finding both Issy and I rather tipsy at 4.15pm on a Wednesday afternoon. To be honest, I think if the circumstances had been different, I would have found his expression rather amusing. Rather peeved, he informed me that he had only come home to change his clothing and that he would then be returning to work as he had been given the opportunity to work extra hours that day.

It was no use; I could contain my emotions no longer. I wrapped my arms around him and cried uncontrollably as I blurted out my terrible news.

"It's true John," Issy confirmed.

Chapter Four

Reality

Now here is something I am sure you will find just as hard to believe as I did, but I think it is important that I share it with you.

As mentioned at the end of the last chapter, John had only come home to change his clothes before returning to work; he had been called out that evening due to bad weather. He worked for our local council and was one of the employees who had put their names forward to work on a winter rota. That meant that if there were any signs of impending snow fall or black ice, he would be called upon to work extra hours gritting surrounding motorways and roads within the area.

Naturally, after hearing the news of my cancer diagnosis, any thoughts of work commitments were placed on the back burner and seemed immaterial. After all, there were plenty of workers just like John, all keen to work extra hours to boost their income. John contacted his line manager at work to inform him that he would be unavailable to work that evening, or any other shifts he had been scheduled to do on an overtime basis. The reaction of John's line manager shocked us both. He informed John that he was unsure if his shift could be cancelled that evening, stating that he would have to get back to him on the matter. You would have thought his line manager would have been sympathetic to our situation and just maybe a bit more supportive. In the end he phoned back and informed John that he had managed to get cover for his shift that evening, but with regard to any other shifts that he had already been delegated, that was a matter he would have to take up with the manager of the depot in which he worked.

That evening was one of the longest I have ever experienced, as well as one of the most intense. John and I talked and cried about our life together and of the dreams we had shared for our future, before being told the awful news of my cancer. John tried his hardest to stay strong for me by constantly reassuring me that everything would be fine, but his words did nothing to make me feel better.

No one telephoned our house that evening, probably due to family and friends not knowing quite what to say, or being too upset themselves.

I thought a great deal about my poor mum and tried to imagine how she would be handling the whole situation. I didn't have to think that hard. Being a mother myself, I could understand my own mother's feelings and it broke my heart knowing that she would now being going through great emotional pain at the possibility of the one thing she dreaded the most. I was overwhelmed by this awful feeling of helplessness at not being unable to take away my mother's pain.

The alcohol that I had drunk earlier had done nothing to deaden my anguish, nor did it make things easier to accept, so in the end I found myself pushing it away in favour of mugs upon mugs of tea. I thought it would make the evening pass more quickly, but it didn't and I found time at a standstill on occasions. When John and I finally made our way to bed in the hope that we would be able to sleep the remainder of the night away, it was impossible. The minute I tried to close my eyes, my mind would run at a million miles an hour with thoughts of my life, my family and death. When I tried to clear my mind of these thoughts, I would find myself thinking of the biopsies I was to have taken the following day. I was so frightened. John also was having great difficulty trying to sleep and in the end we both lay there in the dark not saying a word, too frightened I think to reveal our thoughts to each other.

By 2am, we had both had enough and given that sleep was impossible, we decided to get dressed and go for a walk. As we made our way outside, I remember thinking how very peaceful the night seemed; all the surrounding houses were in darkness and there was almost total silence apart from the sound of the wind and some cars in the distance.

It's very strange how much you change – and how quickly – when faced with death. As I looked up at the sky and clouds above me, I found myself actually taking time to look, rather than just see. Those of us that are blessed with sight constantly go through life looking at the world and everything in it without taking any real time to actually absorb what we're seeing. Clouds for example; I never appreciated just how beautiful and amazing they really are, or ever took the time to wonder how they actually came about until I experienced the possibility of impending death. I am not a philosopher or anything like that, just your normal run of the mill person, but now with a sudden and whole new outlook on the intensity of simple things and their beauty, it was almost as if it was my way of telling my inner self that I had to stay alive in order to now be able to appreciate the things that I had once ignored.

I now believe through my own experiences that everyone faced with death must experience feelings such as these, but I guess I will never know unless I ask someone; maybe I will, one day.

John and I slowly walked hand-in-hand, not really knowing where we were going, or how far we intended to walk; it was as if our brains were incapable of making even the simplest of decisions. In the end, we just went through the motions of putting one foot in front of the other and turned a corner when the notion took us.

Thoughts of my impending biopsies were now making me feel so anxious and I found myself wishing that they were all over. Back in reality, I was beginning to become increasingly angry within myself at the fact that time just dragged on and on. Since walking did not seem to fulfil our need for the night to pass quickly, both John and I therefore decided to turn back and head for home.

As we passed the petrol station at the bottom of our estate, I gestured to John that I wanted to go in. It wasn't as if there was anything particular that I wanted to buy; it was just my way of passing a little more time. Once inside, we both stood scanning the magazine shelves, not really looking, but going through the motions anyway. Eventually, John pick up a few daily newspapers and then we both made our way to the checkout. The woman behind the desk was local and someone we knew. With a strange look, she asked us what on earth we were doing out at that time of night when most folks would be tucked up in bed. Giving a half hearted smile, we both made some remark at not being able to sleep, then quickly left.

Back at the house, the kettle went on for yet another mug of tea. Taking a seat, I tried my best to read one of the papers that John had just bought, but it was impossible; I was totally focused on cancer and no matter how hard I tried, I could not erase these thoughts from my mind.

Time dragged on and it wasn't until around 5am that John and I once again made our way back to bed in the hope that our physical and mental exhaustion would enable us to fall sleep.

Opening my eyes, I felt overjoyed when I looked at the clock on my bedside table and found that it was now 7am. It was almost a relief knowing that at least for an hour and a half I had managed to get some rest from the torment I had experienced. However, these joyful feelings did not last long and before I knew it I was experiencing intense fear at what lay ahead for me that day.

By 8.30am, the pit of my stomach was churning as I showered and dressed in preparation for my visit to the hospital. Yes, I had been desperate for the previous night to end so that I could have the tests I required, but now that morning had arrived, I felt physically sick.

As the front door of our house opened, I realised that it would be my sister Issy. She had wanted to come with us to the hospital that day, something I was glad of because both she and John could be a support for each other whilst they waited.

Getting into our car, I knew that at least we would not have to experience the long wait we had endured the day before; the clinic I was to attend that morning knew I was arriving for in depth biopsies.

As we walked through the corridors of the hospital in the direction of the clinic, I could feel my heart pounding and my panic rising. The clinic was empty when we arrived, apart from the receptionist. Informing her of my reasons for attending the clinic that day, I then made my way to the waiting area of the clinic and took a seat, followed by both John and Issy.

Shortly afterwards, we were joined by Jean, the breast care nurse. She enquired as to how I was feeling, but I think she already knew the answer to her own question by the expression on my face, which most definitely showed the fear that engulfed me. Interrupting her, I introduced her to John and, once again, my sister.

I had many questions that I so desperately needed answered.

"Where are the possible sites of secondary breast cancer?" I found myself asking in a voice tinged with panic.

Jean informed me that there were a few places where secondary breast cancer could rear its ugly head and then went on to list them. Lungs, bones, liver and the brain were all mentioned and I remember thinking how unbelievable her words seemed. Taking a deep breath, I knew I had to ask, "What if I have secondary breast cancer? Would that mean I have less time to live, or could die?"

Given, as I said earlier, that I had been employed in the care industry all of my working life, I had a wide range of knowledge with regard to most medical matters, but none relating to breast cancer.

Jean again began to speak; in a calm voice she informed me that secondary breast cancer could reduce my percentage of life expectancy. Why I asked that question I don't know, because it was clear to me that would be the answer. Perhaps there was a glimmer of hope that she would answer me differently, but it was not to be. Jean did highlight that our discussion was purely hypothetical, whilst also reminding me that my cancer may very well have been diagnosed before it had had a chance to spread to any other organs within my body. Oh how I prayed she was right.

It's strange, but I just kept having these feelings of everything being so unreal and that at any moment someone would come up to me and say that there had been a terrible mix up and I did not have cancer. Alas, that never happened.

Jean rose to her feet informing me that she would be back shortly; she then excused herself and walked in the direction of the consultation room. I wondered what was being discussed behind the scenes by the doctors that I had been scheduled to see that day. Would they be saying that all intervention would be futile as I was destined to die from this tumour that was invading my body, or would they be thinking "Poor soul" and at the same time thanking God that they weren't in my shoes? Would they be disinterested and be viewing the whole situation in a detached manner, as just another part of their job? These were all the thoughts that raced through my head whilst John, Issy and I all sat in silence, waiting on what seemed like a knife edge for someone to call my name.

A few minutes later, the appearance of Jean once again told me instinctively that the doctors were now ready to see me. My heart pounded in my chest as I got to my feet and I felt physically sick as I walked the short distance from the waiting area to the treatment room. My only consolation was that I had this woman by my side to offer the much needed support I now required.

On entering the consultation room, I was met by three doctors; two male and one female. I was asked if I was aware of what procedure I was having done that day. I informed the female doctor that I was and that everything had been fully explained to me the previous day by the doctor. I was then asked if I would remove the upper half of my clothing and put on a hospital gown that lay flat on the chair beside me.

Now alone, screened only from the doctors' view by a curtain that surrounded the examination table, I did as I was instructed. Once gowned up, I pulled the curtain slightly to one side as a way of letting the doctors know that I was ready.

The female doctor spoke first. She asked me to sit upright on the examination table, explaining that by being positioned in this way, a clear access point could be obtained from which to retract the required samples. With the back rest of the table supporting me, I again did as I was instructed, although before giving the doctor the opportunity to begin the procedure, I instantly turned to Jean and asked if she would stand beside me and hold my hand. Saying nothing, she did as I asked.

The female doctor was Australian, I think, with long, wild, flyaway hair. I remember thinking to myself that I would never have guessed that she was a doctor if I had met her under different circumstances. It's strange, but I did feel rather deflated at the fact that it was not the doctor I had seen the previous day who would be performing the tests. Again, the female doctor spoke. This time she explained that she would be taking either three or four tissue samples from the side of my left breast that had been highlighted as cancerous. She then went on to tell me something I would have rather she had kept to herself.

"This procedure can be painful, as numbing deep into the cavity of the breast is difficult."

"Why did she have to share that information with me?" I thought, as I gripped the nurse's hand tighter.

Sitting there upright, with my hospital gown now opened, fully exposing my breasts, I felt totally vulnerable and wished John was the one beside me holding my hand.

The female doctor really did not instil a feeling of ease within me, especially after administering a local anaesthetic to my left breast before proceeding to flaunt the instrument that she required for the procedure directly in front of my face. I do not think for one minute that it was her intention to cause me any distress; I believe she was actually unaware that what she was doing was contributing to my increasing fear.

As I looked at the other doctors that were in the room, it was apparent that they too did not rate the female doctor's bedside manner either. In fact, they looked rather sorry for me, which only added to my anxiety.

The instrument that was to be used to extract the required samples, I would describe as a small metal gun-like contraption, which had a long inner rod coming from where a bullet would travel from the barrel of a real gun. The long rod appeared hollow, with the exception of a pincer like mechanism which grasped the biopsy in a quick, reflex-like manner, as explained to me by the female doctor.

Things seemed to go from bad to worse once the mechanism was inside my breast, for at one point the female doctor appeared to experience difficulty as she tried to manoeuvre the tool in order to obtain the samples she required. As she fiddled and tried to get into the right position, she only seemed to make matters more difficult for herself and, of course, for me.

Again, I looked at the faces of the two male doctors; they now looked as if they were the ones experiencing the procedure themselves. The only thing now in my favour was that the local anaesthetic had in fact been very effective and I felt no pain – and just as well, I remember thinking to myself. At one point, one of the male doctors appeared to become really frustrated by the female doctor's inability to complete the procedure and even gestured that he would take over. However, just at that moment, the gun was in position and the last sample was taken.

I could see by the way the male doctor had reacted that it was for my benefit that he had offered to take matters into his own hands; he appeared genuinely concerned for me and seemed anxious with regard to the time it took the female doctor to complete the procedure. I must admit his actions restored my faith in doctors, something that had been gradually diminishing whilst in the hands of this woman.

Now for those of you who are thinking the worst thoughts imaginable at what this procedure entailed, or now fear the thought of ever having to go through these tests yourselves, please let me once again reassure you that I felt no pain, just slight discomfort, and that the whole process was bearable. I must admit though, I did give a very large sigh of relief when it was all over.

I was informed by one of the doctors that I could go home and that I was not required to return to the hospital again until the day before my surgery in order to have a few blood samples taken prior to my impending operation. The small incisions in my breast were covered by a few basic sticking plasters and I was then left on my own to get dressed.

I would like to mention something, which hopefully will be noted by any doctor who happens to be reading this book. During my procedure, and on more than one occasion, other doctors at the clinic walked into the consultation room in a matter of fact way whilst I was sat on the examination table with the top half of my body openly exposed. Not one of them bothered to knock before breezing into the treatment room and, to add insult to injury, one of them even watched the extracting of my biopsies. I can only hope that it is something that does not happen too often, because the whole experience was rather embarrassing and not very pleasant. Some people don't think, or put themselves in the patient's position, and that's all I will say on the matter.

Cancer No Not Me!

The relief that I felt at knowing now that my ordeal was over was intense. I quickly made my way back to the waiting area where I knew both John and Issy would be waiting anxiously for me to return. Jean remained close by and when she saw that I was about to leave, she made a point of coming over to me and my family to say her goodbyes. I was truly moved by her actions and thanked her for the support that she had given me throughout that morning.

Making our way out of the hospital, I began to tell both John and Issy all about the consultation, as I sighed with relief at knowing that I could now put the whole experience behind me.

Once in our car, John began to drive in the direction of my mum and dad's house. I had not yet seen my mother face to face since being told I had cancer and I desperately wanted to be with her. Truth be told, I just wanted to arrive at her house, run into her arms and cry my heart out, but I knew that was something I wouldn't be doing. I knew I had to be strong and positive for my mum and I also knew she would be composing herself to be strong and positive for me.

I felt sad at knowing that because we do not want to see a person we love in pain, either in a physical or mental sense, we instinctively hold back our true emotions in the hope of making it easier for our loved one to bear the burden that has been thrust upon them.

My mother was standing at her front window waiting for us to arrive. Knowing her as I did, I was sure she would have spent the full morning at that window in anticipation of my return from the hospital. As our car came to a stop outside the house, I could feel the butterflies in my stomach. Once in my mother's house, we both just looked at each other and instantly tears filled our eyes. Giving my mum a big cuddle, I told her not to worry and that everything would be alright.

As we sat close together, I found myself regurgitating words similar to those the consultants had said to me the day before; something about how great advances had been made in the treatment of breast cancer and how it wasn't as life threatening as it had been in years gone by, all in the hope that my words would ease my mother's pain. However, I knew that no matter how much reassurance I tried to give, it would not make a blind bit of difference. What was happening to our family could not be made any easier for any of us, least of all my poor mum.

Time dragged by over the next ten or so days as I waited desperately for my son Billy to return from America. The hardest part of him being so far away was the telephone conversations that we shared. He would telephone and excitedly tell me of all the things he had been doing, update me on all the new friends that he had made and also scare the living daylights out of me by describing in great detail how he lived close to bears; yes real bears.

I remember thinking to myself that the way my luck was going, never seeing my son again would not be because of me dying during surgery, but because of him being killed by a bloody great bear. When voicing my concerns to him about the bears, he just laughed and said, "Don't be silly, I will be alright." Alright? He would never realise just how much I needed him to be alright.

The hardest part of the conversations shared by my son and I were for me to try and remain calm and sound as normal as possible. I would lie through my back teeth that everything was just fine at home and all the while tears would be trickling slowly down my face. When this happened, I would

Cancer No Not Me!

then quickly finish our conversation, telling Billy to enjoy himself and then hand the receiver to John as I went into another room to cry uncontrollably.

During the days and nights before my impending operation, I received loads of cards and flowers from family, friends, work colleagues and neighbours, all expressing how I was in their thoughts and wishing the best for me, actions that were priceless and meant the world to me.

Jean, my breast care nurse, was also becoming a big part of my life. She would often keep in touch with me via telephone to ask how I was coping and to also give reassurance or answer any questions I might have had. A lot of the time, however, when our telephone did ring, I would tell John that I did not want to speak to anyone other than very close family members or Jean. Even then, on a few occasions, I refused to talk to them. After a while, I must say that John became a master of telling little white lies on my behalf, such as, "She's upstairs sleeping", or "She is across at her sister's house". That would be on those occasions when I just couldn't bring myself to speak to anyone. It was at these times I would experience a feeling of complete solitude, where I felt that none of the people I was close to could understand how I was feeling because they did not have cancer.

There were many days when I would find myself just crying endlessly. It was like a blanket of panic that descended over me and no matter how hard I tried to shift these emotions, I found I just couldn't drum up an ounce of positive thinking, only thoughts of impending death. John was my knight in shining armour at these times and would often try to cheer me up by saying things like, "Snap out of it, Roseann; you're going to be alright", or "Stop shedding so many tears over the carpet; you'll ruin it". I think he just said the first thing that came into his head in order to try and distract me from my thoughts. Most times this approach would work and the both of us would have a good laugh at the whole situation.

If ever John had a skill for something, it was making people laugh. The bugger once told me that I obtained a diagnosis of breast cancer just to skive off work. He would also tell me that by being such a strong person I could beat this cancer that was invading my body. Of course, a lot of what he said was in fun; his way of trying to keep my spirits up. He knew I was a very determined person and by teasing me and being honest at times, he could raise my spirits and fuel my determination in my fight to survive. Really quite a clever chap wouldn't you say?

The day of my son's return from America arrived and again that sick feeling in the pit of my stomach returned, together with feelings of relief that I would finally be able to see him. I so desperately wanted to hold him in my arms and tell him how much I loved him. Not that I had any doubts that he didn't know that, but for me it was something I had to tell him face to face, just in case he had forgotten. I know that sounds daft, but I just wanted to roll all the love I had for him since the day he was born into one big "I love you", as truthfully I didn't know how many more chances I would have to say those words. It was also the day before my surgery.

As the car that brought Billy from the airport pulled up outside the house, the atmosphere inside became more and more tense.

"How are you going to tell him? Do you think it's best I leave the room?"

I was throwing these questions at John and answering them myself before he even had the chance to register what

I was saying. "Hell, why does life have to be like this? It's just not fair", I remember thinking.

John and I had talked briefly about how we should tell Billy, but hadn't really come up with a definitive plan. We knew it was going to be hard, but had no answers as to how best to handle the situation; our emotions were just so highly charged. As Billy entered the house, it no longer mattered how we were going to tell him; there was no time left to think any more.

No matter how gently broken, the news was going to be hard to digest, just as it had been for me on that day at the hospital and also for John when he had returned from work later the same day.

Billy entered the living room of our home exhausted and excited from his long journey. He automatically dropped his case at his feet. This was one of the most heart rending situations I had ever experienced. Here was my son, home from his holiday in America, suntanned and full of the joys of life and enthusiastically waiting to tell us all about his dream holiday. All the while he was blissfully unaware of what was about to unfold and how his life was about to change forever.

Momentarily, John and I just stood there watching our son, neither quite sure of what to say or where to begin. John spoke first and started by telling Billy how I had been at the hospital for what we thought would be a run of the mill visit. Slowly he then revealed that it hadn't worked out that way and it was discovered that I had breast cancer. All the while, my son stood frozen to the spot in shock as John continued to tell all that had happened whilst he had been in America. I could feel the tears fill my eyes as I looked at my beautiful son. I was so proud of him. At last I got what I had longed for; to wrap my arms around my baby and tell him how much I loved him.

Billy tried to remain calm and in control, as I knew he would, but the moisture that filled his eyes told me that it was taking every last bit of strength he could muster to remain composed. Like me, he was now the one trying to be strong, not wanting to show how much he was hurting inside.

All the excitement that would normally have come hand in hand with Billy's return would not be shared that day. Instead there was almost an unearthly silence that filled the next few hours as we all tried in our own way to cope with this tragedy that now engulfed our world. To this day, an overwhelming feeling of sadness washes over me as I recall that period of my life.

That evening John and I had made plans to go out for a meal. It was almost like the last supper you could say, but I hoped by doing this it would help the night to pass more quickly.

Nerves had started to build up inside of me at the thought of the major surgery I was scheduled to have the following day. Thoughts that it would most probably be the last day of my life continually haunted me. I tried to appear happy and relaxed for the sake of John and Billy, but it was difficult.

John and I had tried to persuade Billy to join us that evening, but he declined. To be honest, I think he just had to get away from the both of us so that he could openly release his emotions alone, most probably to protect me from any further emotional turmoil.

After telephoning a friend, he asked John if he would drive him over to collect his car, telling us that he would spend some time with his friend before returning home.

On his return, I asked John how Billy had been and what they had talked about whilst alone, but John briefly said

I had nothing to worry about and that our son was fine. However, I knew that this was just John's way of trying to relieve some of the burden that weighed so heavily on me. It was unsuccessful though, because all I could focus on was how my family would survive without me. My heart bled for my parents and I feared that John would be unable to cope on his own. As for my son, the pain he would experience at losing me was too unbearable to imagine. I felt anger, panic and fear at the thought of being robbed of my life and my family.

I was brought back to reality by the sound of John's voice.

"Are you ready?" he asked.

With that, I went through the motions of putting on my coat and shoes and then made my way outside. The place that we had booked for our meal was not that far from where we lived and before I knew it we had arrived at the restaurant and were being shown to a table situated in the corner of the room. I was grateful for that fact because it meant John and I would be able to talk out of earshot of the other people in the room.

I had told John earlier that I was going to order the biggest T-bone steak in the restaurant.

"Well, I don't know when my next meal will be; I have to stock up," I jested.

Normally I would have savoured the thought of a juicy steak, but that evening I had no appetite; nerves made sure of that.

Sitting in the restaurant together, almost alone in our own little isolated corner, I found that gradually I began to relax. At one point John and I even managed a joke about my forthcoming meal making me too heavy for the hospital porters to lift me from one trolley to another.

T-Bone steak at the ready, I was determined to eat as much of it as I could and at the same time made sure for John's benefit that I looked as if I was enjoying every mouthful. I wanted this night to be special. If I was going to die, the last thing I wanted was John's final memory of me to be one plagued with doom and gloom.

We joked about how I would most probably be in no fit state for anything the following day, doped to the eyeballs with pain medication. You might think this is morbid, but it made us laugh; something that we had rarely done over those past few weeks.

Chapter Five

It Was Time

The day of my surgery had arrived; 3 December 1999. Nervously I showered, then double checked the things that I would be taking with me to hospital. Apart from having to go to the hospital the day before my surgery to have blood samples taken, I had not set foot in the place since that memorable day when I had to have further biopsies taken.

At around 7.15am, John and I arrived at the hospital and made our way to the admissions desk. The whole place was deadly silent with only a few hospital staff who appeared to be making their way to their respective departments or the wards to begin their shift for the day.

After checking in, I was informed that I should make my way to the ward. As both John and I walked in the direction of the elevators, I didn't quite know who felt worse; we were like two robots just going through the motions of doing what we were programmed to do.

I tried hard that morning to appear unaffected by what was happening for the sake of John, but the truth of it was that all the while I was terrified.

As we arrived at the ward, we were approached by a nurse who quickly glanced through my paperwork before escorting us into a side room. She stated that she would go and complete my admission details and then return to show me to my bed.

The room we were lead to was empty, apart from ourselves. We took a seat and waited. After a few minutes, the nurse that had been attending to us returned and before I knew it I was standing beside a bed in one of the four-bedded hospital bays within the ward. This was to be my bed for the duration of my stay in hospital.

I quickly glanced around trying to absorb my surroundings. I noted that there was a bathroom within the bay and remember thinking to myself "Thank God", as my nerves were seriously taking over the control of my bladder and I now found I desperately needed to pee.

I didn't look at the other beds, or notice with whom I would be sharing my hospital stay; I was too nervous to be bothered about such things. Taking the seat that was positioned at the side of the bed, I tried to calm my ever increasing nerves, but to no avail. Just as I was about to sit down, a different nurse approached me in a rather hurried manner. She informed me that a porter had arrived to take me to theatre. Honestly; I'm not lying. You could have knocked me down with a feather.

I remember instantly thinking that she must be getting me mixed up with one of the other patients. Not for a minute did I believe she was right in what she said. The nurse then placed a paper pack on the bed informing me that its contents were the cap and gown I would be required to wear in theatre. I just stood there momentarily in sheer disbelief at what was happening to me. Now I really did have to go to the toilet, Telling the nurse this, I began to walk towards the bathroom.

"You will have to be quick," she informed me.

My heart was now pounding at an alarming rate. John and I just looked at each other totally stunned. After returning quickly from the toilet, I then slowly pulled the hospital screens around my bed and began to change as instructed. I never thought I would experience such a feeling of, how can I say it, indignity and lack of control; it was awful.

I had expected that I would have had plenty of time with John before I went to theatre where I would have had the opportunity tell him how much I loved him, even if it was for about the millionth time that morning. Instead, there I was at the point of no return, with no time to waste before I would be whisked away to theatre, robbed of the time I thought I had left to share my deepest feelings with the man I loved. Within a few short minutes John would be leaving the hospital without me, with only a quick goodbye and peck on the cheek. That was one of the most horrible experiences of my life. I just wanted to openly cry, but it would have only distressed John. I had to be brave, so kissing him I told him not to worry and reassured him that everything would be alright. I told him I would see him later that day, all the while praying to myself that the words I had said would come true.

So there I was, all alone, with not even a pre-med drug to help me to relax. My heart was pounding and before I knew it I found myself hopping onto a porter's trolley that was now beside me. By no means ready, but now on my way, I was pushed in the direction of the elevator that would take me to theatre.

As I was wheeled through the hospital corridors with a nurse by my side, I was half hoping that I might see John one last time before he left the hospital, but there was no sign of him. I lay back on the trolley and just looked at the ceiling as I pleaded inwardly to God to let me live through my surgery. My priority was to wake up from my operation; everything else was irrelevant at that point.

Cancer No Not Me!

My mind jolted back to reality as I found that the trolley had come to a halt; we were at the entrance of the operating theatre. Pressing on a keypad that operated the entrance doors to the theatre, the porter – then in continual motion – whisked me into a clinical, ward-like room filled with other beds, all of which I noted were empty. Shouting my name, the porter then brought the trolley to a standstill as he waited for further instructions from one of the theatre staff. All the while the nurse from the ward remained beside me.

Within seconds, two nurses from theatre approached us, double checking my details with the nurse who had escorted me from the ward and both giving me a sympathetic smile as they went about their business. After the formalities, I was asked by one of the theatre nurses to transfer from the trolley onto a theatre bed, which by this time had already been wheeled next to me. Once on this bed, I was then wheeled to join the row of beds that were vacant. I was then left on my own as all of the hospital staff who had been dealing with me disappeared in the direction from which we had all originally come.

So there I was, alone and frightened, with no one to offer support or reassurance, which only added to the intense fear that plagued me. My mind was now racing with all the horrible thoughts I had experienced in the past, but multiplied tenfold. Will I wake up in the middle of my surgery? What if I am aware of what is happening to me, but unable to tell anyone? What if I feel the pain of my surgery, but can't express this to the theatre staff because I am temporarily paralysed by some of the drugs they use during operations?

There is something to be said for pre-meds prior to an operation. If only I had been given one, then at least I believe I would have been spared some of the anxiety.

For those of you out there who are about to, or may ever be faced with impending surgery, make sure that you state firmly that you require a pre-med prior to your surgery. From past experience, I know full well that they make you feel completely relaxed, as though you don't have a care in the world. If given the option, I would take a pre-med every time.

It was time. A nurse clad with theatre gowns walked in my direction. "Oh God, here we go," I thought, as I was then wheeled to another much smaller side room where an anaesthetist waited for me to arrive.

As I was being prepared to visit the land of nod, the door of the room opened and in walked my surgeon, Alison Lanagan. Smiling, she enquired how I was feeling. She clearly couldn't see the fear on my face. My reply to her question was something about not believing it possible to be admitted to hospital and transported to surgery in such a short period of time. I then emphasised how I had wished there had been time for me to have been given some sort of drug to relax me.

Alison informed me that her reasons for taking me so quickly to theatre after my arrival was because she had hoped by doing so she would have spared me increased stress at having to lull about the ward with time on my hands. Once she had explained the reasons behind her rush to get me to theatre, I could appreciate that in her wisdom her actions were for my benefit. Here was a woman who I hardly knew, who was openly considering my personal feelings and genuinely trying to limit my emotional stress. Putting it that way, I could understand the logic behind her plan and even respected her for her thoughtfulness.

To you, Alison, my wonderful surgeon, I would like to share my feelings. I was frightened almost to the point of wanting to scream and would have truly loved a pre-med, if only to relieve me of my mental torment.

In recovery, I remember opening my eyes only to see another set of eyes looking down at me. They were the eyes of the nurse that had been given the responsibility of taking care of me once I had been moved to recovery after my surgery.

"Are you in pain?" she asked.

I only had to nod my head and in an instant the nurse was giving me something to relieve it. That is basically all I recall about my time in recovery. I assume I must have slowly drifted back into a state of unconsciousness. The next time I opened my eyes, I was being transferred from a trolley to my bed in the ward and even then it was only momentary.

I have very little recollection of the rest of that day; it sailed by as one big blur. John did come to see me that evening, but with the effects of the morphine I found it hard to remember much about his visit, although just knowing that he had been by my side for a short period of time that evening meant the world to me.

The remainder of that evening was much the same; one minute I would be awake, but felt exhausted and the next I would look up at the wall clock in the ward amazed by how the time had just flown by.

At one point a couple of nurses came to the side of my bed to assist me with a body wash, something for which I was truly grateful. It felt so good and along with the drugs that I had been given, it contributed to a full night's sleep.

The following morning I felt as if I had been hit by a train and found myself instantly looking for a nurse to request something for my pain. I was so very grateful when a young nurse arrived shortly after to give me my much needed drugs.

I did wonder whether my entire breast had been removed, but I found myself too scared to look down at my body.

As the morning went on, I began to slowly feel more compos mentis. I was sure that the morphine medication I had been receiving had been reduced, because when trying to move even slightly I found I was very sore and tender.

One of the nurses on duty approached me to offer assistance by helping me was a shower. I must admit that although this was something I desperately wanted, I found that I was rather apprehensive, not only worried about the prospect of possibly getting the wound dressing wet, but because I had also noticed that I had two drains protruding from behind my dressings. I was terrified at the thought of the drains being either caught up whilst I was showering, or dislodged in some way. I needn't have worried. Upon explaining my fears to the nurse, I was instantly reassured that all of my worries were unfounded and that she could envisage no problems, explaining that my drains were held in place by small stitches and would definitely not dislodge.

"I will stand beside you, but on the opposite side of the shower screen and hold your drains while you wash," she informed me.

I wish she had known just how much her manner and reassurance had put me at ease.

Preparing to shower, even with the young nurse's help, was a major performance. Exhaustion and the surgery had made it difficult for me to move or raise my arms above my head. By the time I had got my nightdress off, I felt I could quite easily have abandoned all thoughts of showering in favour of returning once again to bed.

Taking a deep breath, I prepared myself to look at my chest. When I did I was surprised and amazed to find that my left breast was still very much apparent. I felt euphoric. I think I would have jumped for joy if it hadn't been for the fact that I had just come through a major surgical procedure. I was elated as I immediately thought that it couldn't have been as bad as my surgeon had first suspected. I couldn't wait to tell my family.

After successfully managing to keep my dressings dry, I then lightly dried myself, still feeling exhausted but much better at having showered and being able to wear one of my own nightdresses.

I slowly made my way back to my bed and asked the nurse if she would bring me the hospital telephone. I could wait no longer. Exhausted as I was, I just had to telephone John with the news that my breast was still intact. Things could only get better.

As I lay on top of my bed, happy at having shared my good news with John, I closed my eyes and tried to get some much needed rest. I must have slept soundly for at least an hour before being woken by the arrival of both Jean and Alison. Alison explained that both she and Jean had visited me the previous afternoon, but that I had been rather groggy. I tried to recall their visit, but could not.

"How are you feeling?" Alison continued.

"Sore," I replied.

She then went on to tell me that as I would now be aware, she had only removed my tumour and the lymph nodes from under my left armpit.

"Your surgery went well," she reassured me.

She then went on to explain that with regard to any further treatment that I might require, we would have to wait for the results from the analysis of both my tumour and lymph nodes before any decisions could be made. With nothing further to add, she and Jean said their goodbyes.

"All I can do now," I told myself "is concentrate on getting better." Thank goodness things weren't as bad as I had originally thought.

The rest of my stay in hospital was made so much easier by a friendship that I had struck up with a fellow patient; he had also been diagnosed with having cancer. Tom was about eight years older than me and had been diagnosed with stomach cancer.

As I had mentioned earlier, you do seem to experience a bond with others that have, or have had cancer. Maybe the fact that there was someone who knew exactly how I was feeling had something to do with it. I know from my friendship with Tom that the understanding, respect and more importantly the truth we got from each other, gave great comfort. I no longer felt alone; here was someone just like me, travelling on an emotional rollercoaster with no crystal ball to give even the slightest clue as to what lay ahead.

We were each able to discuss many issues with no holds barred; family, finances, fear of death and innermost secrets if you like, all spoken with mutual understanding. It was almost like having a twin, a mirror image of how one feels to have been diagnosed with cancer. Although we were both diagnosed with cancer in two totally different areas of our bodies, that made no difference; cancer was our common bond.

I considered myself blessed during that stay in hospital in that I had Tom as a friend. We would speak for hours, sometimes into the night or even during it when we both found sleep impossible. We were just there for each other, almost like a crutch. We would tell each other all about our lives and families and on some occasions even shared a giggle.

I think it's sad these days that financial cutbacks have taken their toll on the field of medicine. People with all different illnesses are now all thrown together into one ward, like eggs in a basket. When that happens, there is a great feeling of isolation. You can't understand how the person in the next bed to you is feeling. How can you when you have both been admitted for two totally different operations for two totally different illnesses? That is the way I felt until I met Tom, my fellow cancer sufferer, a few days after my surgery.

After we were both discharged from hospital, we remained in touch for some time, although half the time we would be scared to telephone each other. You see we always shared the fear that on one of the occasion that we picked up the telephone, it would be only to hear the news we dreaded, that one of us had received news that our cancer had returned. During the telephone conversations that we did have, we would often talk about the experience we felt at not feeling like the same person we once were before having cancer. We would also comment on the restrictions that we now experienced. For instance, I had very little power in my left arm and Tom was only able to eat very small portions of food at any given time.

I returned home less than a week after my surgery. There was nothing else for me to do other than concentrate on my recovery and, once again, play the waiting game.

Only when the tests had been completed on my tumour and lymph nodes would I know what my future held.

Chapter Six

Struggling

It was great to be home. Mentally I was in good form, or so I believed, focusing on the fact that I had not required a full mastectomy, rather than negative aspects. Physically, however, my recovery was slow. The pain I had experienced prior to leaving hospital, which was slight and under control with medication, had now started to increase. It got so bad at times that it would literally bring tears to my eyes and would prevent me from obtaining a full night's sleep. On other occasions, the pain would have me pacing the floor and all the pain relief medications I took were ineffective. Sometimes John would walk directly behind me massaging my shoulders in an attempt to try and make me feel better, but even that didn't help.

More often than not, I was finding that I would bite John's head off, not because of anything he had done, but because of the way I was feeling. It was so very hard trying to cope with the pain and lack of sleep. I didn't know what was going on inside my body physically, but what I did know was that things were getting worse instead of better.

A few days after my return from hospital, John said, "You can't continue to go on like this."

He picked up the telephone receiver and handed it to me.

"Call the doctor or I will Roseann."

Now you may be wondering to yourself why I hadn't telephoned my doctor before things had got so bad. I suppose I believed that the doctors who were now involved in my care would be well aware of how my recovery would proceed, so with that in mind I was sure that any pain relief medication prescribed when I was discharged from hospital would eventually build up in my system and increase in effectiveness.

Fear also played part in my reluctance to contact a doctor; I was terrified that I would have to go back into hospital, or even worse, that my cancer had spread.

On speaking to the receptionist at our doctor's surgery, she informed me that it was a new practice doctor who was dealing with any telephones queries. With that, she took my details and told me that the doctor would return my call as soon as possible.

Within only a matter of minutes our telephone rang. John handed the receiver to me whilst miming that it was the doctor. As I took the receiver and began to speak, I could feel my emotions heighten and almost instantly began to cry. God only knows what this poor doctor on the other end of the telephone must have thought.

I updated the doctor on the problems I had been experiencing since being discharged from hospital and between sobs told him how the pain medication wasn't working and that I was also having great difficulty sleeping.

"Please can you give me something to ease my pain and help me sleep?" I asked him, as all the while I paced the floor with John right behind me massaging my shoulders.

After hearing the difficulties that I had been experiencing, the doctor was sympathetic and without hesitation informed me that he would write a prescription for stronger painkillers and something to help me sleep. After informing me that my prescription would be ready in about half an hour, he ended the conversation. I think if I had been right beside him at that moment I would have kissed his feet! The relief I felt at knowing that I would soon have something to take away my pain was like a huge weight being lifted from my shoulders.

Once John had collected my new medication and returned home, I not only took the stronger painkillers, but also one of the sleeping tablets. I just had to shut down, because I was physically and mentally exhausted. I really didn't care that it was only late morning as long as what I had taken would rid me of the pain and enable me to sleep. Helped by John, I made my way to bed.

I was surprised when I awoke to find that it was late evening. I couldn't believe that I had slept that long; it was a great feeling knowing not only had I been able to sleep, but it was pain free.

Pain is a funny thing; your mind keeps telling you that surely it's not possible to experience something so severe and at times you even start to doubt yourself. You begin to wonder if all that you are feeling is in your imagination. At times I was beginning to think that I was going off my head, so for those of you out there who are in pain, don't try to battle through it and suffer in silence like I stupidly did. Pain and sleeplessness can, in most cases, be treated by your doctor, something that I now realise. I also now believe that pain causes great stress, so with that in mind it is easy to understand that with these two symptoms combined, your body is not given the chance to heal itself.

Over the days that lead up to my next appointment at the breast cancer clinic, time dragged. The waiting game was almost as bad as the diagnosis and the surgery. I tried to remain positive whilst I waited for my results, focusing yet again on the fact that my left breast had not been removed. I did begin to experience a nagging doubt at the back of my mind triggered mainly by my ongoing pain; my new painkillers had worked for a few days, but were now of no use.

There was no gradual getting better by the day for me; it just didn't happen. I had also now begun to experience difficulty with my left arm. No matter how hard I tried, I found I was unable to fully stretch it out or lift it very high; something I might add my mother would comment on continually, telling me that I had to keep moving and exercising it otherwise it would permanently seize up. She would get my sisters to nag me about it. I would really get frustrated, if not angry at times, when she hounded me. On more than one occasion I snapped my mother's head off, telling her I was trying my best to move my arm but no matter what I did it would not budge. The last thing I needed was someone, even if it was my mum, on my back about it, especially as this was one of the things that was concerning me.

John's mum was another source of grief to me at times. She lived alone as John's dad had passed away about 11 years earlier. When John and I visited her, she would constantly go on about how she had been diagnosed with breast cancer some years previously. She would say, "I've come through it too, you know, and look at me now; I'm fine," but her words just weren't true. She had never in her life been diagnosed with any form of cancer. I often wonder why she said those things to me. Even when I told her that she was talking nonsense, she would still insist in making my life a misery by going on about it. I would get so upset over it and at one stage told John that if he didn't have a word with his mother, then I wouldn't be going back to visit.

I never really fathomed out why she would say these things. Maybe she felt threatened, or even jealous of the intense attention I was receiving from John. Who knows? It could have been her way of trying to reassure me that people can beat cancer. However, whatever her reasons were, the impact of her words aggravated me.

My thoughts would take total control of me at times. I had once watched a programme on television about a young mother who had been diagnosed with breast cancer, which was so very, very sad. I can remember watching her and listening to her words of, "If there is anything that comes from this documentary today, I would want it to be that the women out there look at me and think, 'I will make sure I check my breasts for lumps'". She then went on to say how, like most of us, she had seen a similar programme some years prior to her diagnosis and had thought to herself, "I will make sure I check my breasts for lumps". Again, like most of us, she became complacent; too late in her discovery of a lump to save her life.

That day after watching that programme, I said the exact same thing, that I would make sure from that day on that I checked my breasts regularly for lumps. However, just like that poor woman, it was only words and I stupidly never did really pay much attention to my breasts. It wasn't until pain and discomfort forced me to attend my GP that my diagnosis eventually reared its ugly head.

So please don't be like the young woman who sadly died, leaving two children motherless, or me; check your breasts regularly. Whilst in the bath is an ideal time; you are alone and relaxed and remember, it only takes a few minutes and those few minutes can save your life.

I was told by one of my breast care doctors that one of the best ways of examining your breasts whilst in the bath or during a shower, is to work up a good lather all over your chest and slowly examine each breast lightly with your fingertips in small circular motions.

Cancer No Not Me!

It can also happen to men too. If you don't examine your breasts already, start from today; it just may save your life.

15 December arrived; the day of my appointment. John and my sister Issy attended with me. As we arrived at the hospital and made our way to the breast cancer clinic, I felt rather flat. The clinic was absolutely mobbed with people, with not a spare seat to be found. After checking in at the reception desk, John, Issy and I stood against a wall and waited for some seats to become vacant.

Looking at all the people waiting to be seen, I could now recognise and pick out more often than not the individuals who, like me, had been diagnosed with breast cancer. I suppose one of the tell-tale signs could have been the fact that the people who were not familiar with the clinic seemed to constantly moan about the time it was taking for them to be seen by a doctor. I was never one of them. Others like me that had been diagnosed with cancer were just so grateful that there was a doctor there that could help us. Another sign is the way that cancer sufferers seem to give a smile to all those waiting to be seen, something that the un-diagnosed or cancer free individuals seem to barely register, or even notice at all. The smile is an unspoken symbol of understanding and a way of saying "I hope your treatment's going well", or "You'll get there". It's as if it's our way of saying that we have been given a second chance, or are just grateful that we are still here. Something to do with looking at the world differently, I believe.

Some chairs became available so John, Issy and I all quickly took a seat before they could be filled by anyone else. We then all sat in anticipation as we waited to be seen and told the outcome of the tests on both my tumour and lymph nodes.

"Roseann Gallagher!"

My name was being called. Automatically, both Issy and I walked in the direction of the treatment rooms as John followed behind. On entering the room, I was so very glad to see Alison Lanagan. We had instantly clicked since our first meeting, even though it had been under difficult circumstances. The rapport that had begun to develop between us instilled a feeling of confidence in me. I felt that if anyone could get me through my battle with cancer she could and, if not, I believed that she would give her all in trying.

Jean, my breast care nurse, was also present and I felt pleased to see her. She had been a great support to me and at times I don't know how I would have coped some days without her regular telephone calls.

"How have you been keeping since your surgery?" Alison asked.

There was no stopping me as I launched into great detail about how things had not been great, emphasising that the pain I was experiencing in my left breast was almost intolerable. I also told her about the problems I had been having with my left arm and how I had very little power and movement. Alison nodded her head as if in acknowledgment. It was almost as if she knew beforehand that these were the problems that I would be experiencing.

Looking directly at me, she then went on to tell me how the results from the tests on both my tumour and lymph nodes were not good; words that totally shocked me as I thought, "This isn't possible". If that had been the case, then surely I would have been given a total mastectomy?

All the feelings that I had experienced on that first day when told of my cancer came flooding back. I was once again very frightened. In my mind I was like a headless chicken running about from here to there and not quite knowing where to go. It was as though I was searching for a way out of the situation I now found myself in. John gripped my hand tightly, but I felt no comfort from it. There was no way he could take away my pain or make me feel confident that things would be alright. Issy just sat in total disbelief at what we were being told.

Alison continued, "There is unstable tissue in your breast that would eventually turn cancerous if not removed."

I tried to digest what she was saying, but no sooner had I taken in the terrible news than I was struck a further blow.

"There is also cancer invasion of your lymph nodes."

Everyone remained silent as Alison slowly began to tell me that I would not only require further surgery, but that this time I would have to have a radical mastectomy.

"You may also require a course in radiotherapy," she added.

"Oh God!" I thought, "This is it; I am most certainly going to die."

During the rest of my consultation things just seemed to go from bad to worse. I was told that I would also require further tests to see if my cancer had spread to other areas within my body. I felt numb. I would require an ultrasound of my liver and a chest x-ray, both of which would to be done that day. I was also told I would also require a bone scan, although this could not be arranged for that day. My surgeon did stress, however, that she would request this scan as urgent.

All the while I uncontrollably squeezed John's hand harder and harder. I remember thinking to myself, "This is just not fair. I'm not a bad person. If anything, I would go out of my way for others."

The conversation was then turned to a discussion about my next clinic appointment.

"The results of your further tests, bone scan and liver ultrasound should be completed by then," Alison told me.

"Another bloody waiting game," I remember thinking to myself.

Dates for my next surgery were also mentioned, with 7 January being chosen as the date on which I would once again return to theatre. Things to me were now beginning to make sense with regard to my increased pain and slow recovery. No wonder I had all these problems; if the tissue in my breast was unstable then obviously my body's healing processes would be affected. On realising this, I asked Alison if she would prescribe me another form of pain relief. If I was pain free, at least that would be something.

I also thought, "Well if that was the bloody case, then why the hell was my breast not removed during my last operation?" something I did voice to Alison. She did give me a full explanation, but to be honest it didn't register in my head; there were too many things floating about in there already.

Now you may think I'm mad to say this, but the good thing that did come out of that day was that yet again I could go into hospital on the actual day of my surgery. I think Alison felt that I needed something to go in my favour and for that I was grateful.

Again, I walked through the corridor to the x-ray department. The last time I had made my way there was on the day of my cancer diagnosis. That was where I had been sent to have a mammogram. All those raw emotions resurfaced and feelings of helplessness again overwhelmed me. I was relieved when my name was called rather quickly; I couldn't wait to get out of that place and away from my awful memories.

With my chest x-rays over and done with, I made my way to the ultrasound department, all the while followed by John and Issy. This test entailed lying on a hospital examination table whilst part of my stomach, side and back were then covered in a gel. I then had, what felt like, a ball on the end of a wire rolled around the areas of my body where images of my liver could be viewed and recorded, very similar to an ultrasound given to pregnant mothers, I imagine.

Whilst I was having this test done, I found myself closely watching the face of the doctor doing my scan, hoping I might been able to gauge some sort of expression that would tell me whether the visual results of my liver were good or bad. I needn't have bothered though, for it was as if the doctor had been taught how to remain expressionless, no matter what the outcome.

Once the test had been completed, I did try to get the doctor to tell me what he had seen on the screen, but it was a waste of time; he wasn't for discussing it and would only say that my results would be sent to the doctor that had requested the test.

During the run up to Christmas, I was feeling like shit. My pain did subside slightly with the start of the medication my surgeon had prescribed, but it was always there. Lying down seemed to help on occasions, but then I would experience tremendous discomfort; it was terrible. I also felt totally exhausted all the time and had no real interest in anything, with the exception of my forthcoming surgery. I was beginning to spend most of my time wishing that day would arrive, if only to take away the pain I was experiencing.

Movement in my left arm remained limited and again my mother would be on my back about the importance of keeping it mobile. I would still find myself biting my mother's head off when she brought the subject up.

More often than not, the only thing that kept me sane was the fact that I could gain total relief from my pain and discomfort most of the time when I popped a sleeping tablet into my mouth before bed each evening.

I probably shouldn't admit this, but sometimes I would feel so bad that the only way I could get through the day was to go to bed in an afternoon and take yet another sleeping tablet. However, it was something I did not do on a regular basis, only on the occasions when things were at their very worst.

A few days after my clinic appointment, I received a letter in the post informing me of time and date for my bone scan. The information leaflet that came with my letter explained that my tests would take some hours and it would therefore be an all day appointment. I had to be at the hospital bright and early and the letter stressed that there were definitely no facilities for family members, which made me feel uneasy, as I didn't relish the thought of having to face the entire experience alone.

When the day arrived, John drove me to the hospital and stayed with me in the waiting area of the Nuclear Medicine department until my name had been called. He then gave me a quick kiss, telling me to telephone him when my tests had been completed. My stomach now was doing cartwheels. I felt so very helpless and alone.

In the leaflet I had received with my appointment letter, it explained fully what would happen before, during and after my scan. There was no mention about the test being painful, but nevertheless this gave me no sense of relief, for neither had it mentioned that the procedure would be painless.

Slowly, I walked to the other end of the clinic corridor as instructed, all the while apprehensive about what lay ahead.

I felt almost relieved at arriving, only to find that I had entered yet another smaller waiting area within the clinic. Other than myself, there was a man in a wheelchair with a nurse as his escort. I remember taking the time to look at him in more depth, almost as if to try and ascertain how ill one would have to be in order to require such a test, but was unable to come to any conclusions.

I picked up a magazine from a table in the centre of the room and began to flick through it. Why, I do not know, because I was far too nervous to concentrate on any form of reading material. I suppose it was just one of those things we instinctively find ourselves doing whilst sitting in hospital waiting areas.

When my name was finally called, I was instructed by one of the clinic nurses to come forward and take a seat in a room, not far from where I was sitting. Now with my full attention, the nurse explained to me that in the first instance I would be given an injection in my arm that contained a small amount of radioactive fluid. I was then informed that I would be taken to the clinic dayroom where I would be required to drink between 2–3 jugs of water or juice. The reason behind this was that by passing copious amounts of fluids through my body, I would send the contents of my injection through my system; in other words, the more I drank and passed, the better the scan quality.

After explaining that the whole process would take approximately five hours, the young nurse then escorted me to the clinic dayroom. After the appropriate five hour time period had elapsed, I was then shown to another room; this was where my tests would be completed.

Introducing himself, the man in the room explained that he would be doing the actual scans that I required and that they would be done in stages; head and neck, torso and so on.

"It's nearly over now. After this you will be free to go."

How grateful I was to hear those words. I was so desperately in need of my painkillers, which I had stupidly left at home.

I had assumed that I would have to change into a hospital gown, but to my surprise I was told that there was no need; the only things I was required to remove were my items of jewellery, much to my relief.

Some of the scans were conducted whilst I was lying down and others whilst I was standing. All the while I looked in amazement at the assortment of large machines and computer software contained in this one room; it was all very high-tech.

I could see my body image on one of the monitors and given that I was familiar with the term "hot spots", another expression for cancer spread, I looked intensely at the screen to see if I could identify any. God only knows why I did this, because truthfully, I really didn't have a clue what I should be looking for.

At one point I remember thinking, "Well if hot spots are identifiable by the colour red, then I'm done for", because large areas of my body shown on the screen appeared to have very prominent red patches. Fear began to overpower me again, as I found myself turning my eyes in the direction of the radiographer in the hope of getting a reassuring expression from his face. Extracting nothing from this man's demeanour, I enquired whether there were any signs of cancer. A waste of time really, for his reply was similar to the statement that I had received whilst having my liver scan.

All in all it took about three quarters of an hour for all my scans to be completed. After that it was a matter of waiting for John to come and pick me up and take me home.

I tried hard to sound enthusiastic about Christmas, but the truth is that I wasn't in the least bit interested. Even when it came to presents, I just got a bundle of Christmas cards and added money to them; there was just no way that I could have focused on what present to get and for whom. Now that felt strange, as normally I would have great fun shopping for presents and would spend hours searching for just the right present to match the person. I often giggled away to myself as I searched for that special gift, one that would either give the recipient a good laugh, or one I knew the person especially wanted. Then with all my presents wrapped and under the tree, I would become increasingly excited as Christmas Day drew closer.

Normally, I would be desperate to open my presents on Christmas Eve on the stroke of midnight and John would always go on about how presents were for opening on Christmas morning. So, to keep him happy, I would reluctantly bide my time 'til morning. However, as a way of getting the last laugh – and because I loved doing it – I would make sure that I woke both John and Billy up bright and early as I blasted Christmas songs on our stereo. It was great – a true feeling of Christmas!

Christmas 1999 was different. I found myself uninterested in anything due to the pain and discomfort I was experiencing. It took me all of my strength just to muster a smile. I felt awful. I had no interest in presents and happy faces and truthfully cannot remember what my gifts were that year.

So there I was on Christmas morning, miserable and wishing I could just crawl into a hole until all the celebrations were over. I just wanted to be left alone, but I knew that would not happen. John's mum was coming to our house for Christmas. Billy was a fireman, so he would be on duty, although we would see him at some point in the day. As for our two granddaughters, they always spent Christmas Day with their mum, so as like previous years it would be Boxing Day before we would see them. However, we did listen to them on the telephone as they excitedly told us of all the things they had received from Santa. My own mum and dad were having Christmas dinner with Issy and her family and my other sisters and their families would all be meeting up at some point that evening at Issy's house. My only sister who wouldn't be there was Janet and her family, who now lived in England.

John did everything that day, from picking his mum up to preparing and making the Christmas dinner. As I watched him trying so very hard to make sure that everything was just right, I remember thinking just how much I loved him.

Reluctantly, I walked in the direction of my sister's house with John and his mum. As we entered the house, you could sense the happiness that filled the air; it was obvious that everyone was enjoying themselves. John's mum had been so excited at the thought of spending Christmas Day with us as she got on well with all of my family.

After all the traditional Merry Christmas kisses, I signalled to my mum to follow me into another room. Now this was one present I do remember giving. When we were alone, I handed her a box and told her to open it. Inside I had placed the first ring that John had ever bought me. I wanted my mum to have it as a special Christmas present from me. It was something that I treasured and I knew it would mean the world to my mum. When she saw what was in the box, tears filled her eyes.

"I can't take this," she told me.

But I needed her to, as I wanted so very much to give my mother something of mine that she could treasure, should I die.

"I wanted to give you a very personal gift this year," I told her as I give her a great big cuddle. "I love you mum."

"I love you daughter," she replied.

At that, we both made our way back to join the rest of our family. It felt so good as I watched my mother lightly touch the ring that was now on her finger as if it were a part of me she held in her hand.

Everyone talked of the presents they had received that year and, as the day went on, more members of our family gradually appeared. The children were having a great time, as was John's mum, who was totally engrossed in conversation with my mother. The rest of the family happily mingled with each other. As with most family gatherings, the camera never stopped flashing. Not long after, I told John that I was going home to lie down as it was all getting too much for me. Thankfully, we only lived across the road.

On hearing what I had planned to do, Issy insisted that I go to her bedroom and lie down rather than be alone, so just to please her, I reluctantly did as she suggested. Entering the room, I gave a sigh of relief, glad at the fact that I no longer had to keep up the pretence that all was well. As I lay down on the bed, I began to feel relieved by the peace, even though I could still hear my family laughing and joking in the distance.

For ages, I tried to get myself into a comfortable position, but it was no use; I just could not settle. Close to tears, I decided that the only place I would be able to get comfortable was in my own bed, so after pulling myself up I made my way back to say my goodbyes to my family and then returned home.

It's amazing how intolerant you become to noise when you are in pain. Even trying to hold a conversation with someone becomes difficult; you are unable to focus on what the other person is saying. You then find yourself becoming irritated by that person, not because of them personally, but because of the way you feel. I found that when my pain was at its worst, I could not tolerate any sound at all, even music. It would almost drive me to the point of insanity. It's true; pain gets you like that.

How I managed to get through Boxing Day I will never know. Both Rebecca and Nicola our grandchildren had arrived and were so very excited. Boxing Day at our house is like a second Christmas Day to them, because it's the day when they receive all their presents from their dad and from the rest of our side of family.

When it was time for them to receive their presents from John and me, they truly surprised me by how happily they received our gift of a card each with money in it. I had honestly thought they would have been disappointed. Usually they would receive a large array of gifts from us and I had worried that they would have been disappointed that year, but no. They gave John and I each a great big kiss then happily returned to open the rest of their presents. The house was buzzing with the excited laughter of the girls as they opened one present after the other.

John again had made the meal and I had great fun watching Rebecca as she tried all the different kinds of food on the table. Nicola, however, would have nothing other than chicken nuggets; I was sure that one day she would turn into one!

I did feel tired and at times pain would wash over me, but all in all I got through the day successfully, which pleased me. After all, the last thing I wanted was to spoil the girls' special day, but I have to admit that I wasn't complaining when the time came for them to go home. By then I was totally exhausted and was fit only for bed.

During the days prior to my next clinic appointment, I would periodically go through feelings of doubt with regard to my liver and bone test results. Up to that point, everything seemed to have gone from bad to worse and I was beginning to believe that my life would soon be over. I was feeling just like that on the evening I had arranged for Maggie, my boss and friend, to come and visit. I had not seen her since first taking sick leave and was really looking forward to hearing all the usual work gossip, hoping that it would divert my attention away from all the morbid thoughts that were invading my mind.

John knew Maggie well as we had all been out on a few occasions after work and that comforted me. I knew that if I needed to go to bed, I could quite easily do so as John and Maggie would have been happy to carry on talking away to each other into the wee small hours.

As the night continued, our discussion moved to the subject of my chest x-rays, bone scan and liver ultrasound. Totally out of the blue, I began to cry uncontrollably, blurting through my tears that I knew I was going to die. No amount of reassurance from either John or Maggie would make me believe otherwise. I just fell deeper into a severe bout of depression and I could see no way out. I must have cried for a solid hour before I eventually calmed down and by then I was that totally exhausted.

Alcohol, I believe, had a lot to do with making me feel the way I did that night; the more the alcohol took effect, the more emotional I became. I promised myself that there would be no more over indulging in alcohol for me. I didn't think I could have coped with ever experiencing another night like that one.

Chapter Seven

Swings and Roundabouts

29 December finally arrived; the day I would receive my test results. John had taken me to the clinic that day and thinking back, I can't recall why my sister did not come with us. Maybe it had all become too much for her, or maybe she felt that John and I needed some space.

On entering the consultation room, I could feel the butterflies whizzing around in my tummy as I took a seat and anxiously waited for Alison to speak.

"Good news," she said. "Your chest x-rays and the scans of both your liver and bones show no evidence of cancer," she added.

To say I was relieved would be an understatement. "At last some good news," I told myself.

The fact that I no longer had ovaries, having undergone a hysterectomy some years previously, was also good news. My surgeon explained that all hormone production from this part of my body was now eradicated. Given that the type of cancer I had been diagnosed with was 90% hormone receptive was great news. I was over the moon.

I was jogged back to reality by Alison's voice. Again I listened intently.

"With regard to your admission for your next surgery, I'm afraid that the arrangements for you to be admitted that morning have now been changed. Our anaesthetist has said that he would prefer it if you came into hospital on the evening prior."

I didn't care that I had to be in hospital a day earlier than I had first anticipated. I was just so happy with the news that I had received that day that I don't think anything could dampened my spirits. I just couldn't wait to get home that day to tell my son and the rest of my family. I was so very excited.

Billy was as ecstatic as I was when I told him my good news and when I told my mum I could almost feel her body relax with relief. Everyone else showed the same reaction when I telephoned them. It was indeed a great day.

I spent most of New Year's Eve in bed. I only got up at around 11pm, more for the sake of John than anything else. His face lit up as I walked into our lounge.

"How are you feeling?" he asked.

Giving him a kiss on the cheek I told him I was much better, but that was a lie. As my next surgery date began to draw nearer, I could feel myself become more despondent at the prospect of having to endure further surgery. The way I felt is hard to explain. Yes, I was desperate for the pain to go away, but the closer the date of my surgery came, the more anxious I was. Coping was definitely becoming harder for me, almost to the point at times of feeling that I could take no more.

John brought a smile to my face as I watched him excitedly dash around preparing a drink for us both to welcome in the New Year. He then attempted to coax our dog Tess to join him outside. I laughed as I watched Tess look at John as if to say, "It's bedtime; I'm not going out there", but with little choice, she did.

As I sat alone for a few minutes, I wondered whether I would be alive the following year. I desperately wanted to believe that I would, but even when I tried to tell myself that with no secondary cancer detected things could only get better, the nagging thought of doubt would emerge once again.

With the ringing of our door bell I was jolted back to reality. Opening the front door, John instantly wished me a Happy New Year, whilst Tess ran around excitedly.

John and I spent the next hour wishing all our family members a Happy New Year via telephone. Once we had spoken to everyone, we then sat listening to music as we talked of our hopes for a better year.

Two days before my surgery, my nerves began to rise. I had also begun to feel rather weepy. I just could not believe I had to go through all this again. I had suggested to John that we go out for a meal, just as we had done prior to my previous hospital admission, hoping that by doing so it would take my mind off bloody hospitals, even if it was only for a short time.

As we approached the restaurant, I began to wonder if my suggestion had been such a good idea. Like before, I didn't much feel like eating anything. I tried to tell myself that once I had a meal in front of me then I would feel differently, but even the thought of food made me feel physically sick. I continued walking, not wanting to share with John how I was really feeling. He had enough on his plate.

Once in the restaurant, I ordered the same meal that I had on our last visit; T-bone steak, whilst John ordered a curry. When our order arrived, it looked and smelt delicious, but even that could not tempt me to eat. All I wanted to do was go home and be in my own surroundings. "Poor John," I thought. "He must feel that half the time he does not know if he is coming or going, due to the emotional rollercoaster I put him through at times."

Seeing John look in my direction, I tried for his sake to eat some of the food that was on my plate, but it was no use; it was taking all my time to try and swallow the smallest of portions, let alone eat the whole meal. At that, I began to wrap my steak in my napkin. If I couldn't eat it then Tess would be having a lovely steak for her dinner that night. All the while John looked on. He knew exactly what I was doing; my actions even brought a smile to his face. I felt comfort in knowing that John understood and hadn't made a big thing about it. He knew me so well.

Returning home to a very happy doggie, who thought it was her birthday when I showed her what I had in store for her, almost made my visit to the restaurant worthwhile.

John and I both took a sleeping tablet that night; there was just no way we would have got any sleep otherwise.

On arriving at the ward the following morning, I gave my name to the first nurse I saw and explained that I was due to be admitted that day. The nurse looked sympathetic when hearing my name; it was as if she was fully aware that this would be the second time within five weeks that I would again be going to theatre. I remember thinking that she had most probably read my notes. Again, I was lead in the direction of a four-bedded bay in the ward and shown which bed would be mine whilst in hospital.

The nurse informed me the anaesthetist who had insisted that I be admitted the day before my surgery had already been on the telephone enquiring as to whether I had arrived or not.

"I will contact him now and let him know that you are here," she said.

After changing into a light pair of joggers and t-shirt, I emptied the remainder of my bag, then sat on the bed near to the chair in which John had been sitting. I felt pretty down and voiced this to him.

"You'll be alright," he said reassuringly.

We talked for a while about our family and whether or not the surgery would solve all of my problems. When it was time for John to go, I walked him to the elevator, kissing him and saying that I would phone him later that night and then he was gone.

I hated the feeling of total vulnerability. Oh how I wished that my surgery was over. I sat on my bed, half-heartedly sifting through the magazines that I had brought in with me. I didn't feel in the mood for talking to anyone, so kept my head low in order to prevent me from making eye contact with the other female patients in the bay, who by then were in jovial conversation with each other.

Not long after, a young man approached me and introduced himself by his first name, telling me that he was the bad doctor, responsible for me having to come into hospital a day earlier than originally planned. I jokingly ticked him off. He explained that he had come to take samples of my blood as it was required prior to surgery. I wondered if that meant just in case I needed a blood transfusion. I am not the type of person that is frightened of needles, so I wasn't that bothered. However, when it became more and more obvious that he was not having any luck obtaining blood samples, I began to become slightly anxious, especially when he suggested taking a sample of blood from my leg. This is where he did eventually obtain the required samples.

I think the whole experience was most definitely made easier by the fact that all the while this doctor continued to make small talk as he busily went about the job in hand. If it hadn't been for that, I think my anxiety would have been far worse.

The day of my surgery arrived, along with the butterflies. I quickly showered and waited to be told what would happen next. The day before I had been so caught up with blood samples that I had completely forgotten to mention that I wanted to be prescribed a pre-med. "You silly cow," I told myself. I looked anxiously around for a nurse, hoping to speak to someone about it. With the anaesthetist being so adamant that he wanted me admitted a day earlier than planned, I hoped this meant that he was double checking that he had taken all procedures into consideration.

I managed to catch the attention of one of the nurses and anxiously asked her if she knew when I would be given a pre-med and also if she could tell me what time I had been scheduled to go to theatre. I might as well have been talking to a brick wall; the only response she would give me was a blank look followed by a quick response of, "I will find out for you". With that she disappeared. I had no choice other than to sit and wait for the nurse to return, hopefully with a pre-med.

I watched as staff handed out breakfasts, but of course, none of them were for me. As two of the three patients who were sharing the four-bedded bay with me happily tucked into their cereal, roll and beverage, I noticed that the other patient, an elderly lady, just sat in her bed staring into space. Her tray lay on a bedside trolley situated at the end of her bed, but no one had bothered to move the food nearer to this small frail woman. After a few minutes, and as she appeared slightly confused, I approached her, irritated by the fact that everyone else seemed to be turning a blind eye. On asking her if she would like some breakfast, she instantly replied, "Yes". Honestly, I don't think she knew that the food at the bottom of her bed was for her.

How could the other patients ignore this poor wee soul? I hoped my actions would in some way embarrass them, but they didn't. After taking the time to place the bedside trolley beside the elderly patient, I milked her cereal, buttered her roll and after asking her what she took in her tea, then prepared it for her. I just couldn't believe that neither the other patients nor any of the nurses had taken a couple of minutes to help this frail old lady. I am a great believer in small acts of kindness and thoughtfulness meaning a lot, but obviously it seemed I was the only one. It angered me knowing that the nursing staff were more familiar with this woman than I, so should have known she would not be able to sort out her breakfast without a little bit of help.

Returning to my bed, I watched as this old woman happily tucked into her breakfast. It concerned me to think that on other occasions this old lady most likely went without because she was not given the help she obviously needed.

The nurse to whom I had spoken earlier returned to inform me that I would be going to theatre shortly and handed me the now familiar theatre pack containing both a gown and cap.

"What about my pre-med?" I almost screeched at her.

"Nothing was mentioned about a pre-med," she said.

As I watched her walk away, I just sat there in sheer disbelief at what she had just told me. It was happening all over again. I could feel the tears begin to build up in my eyes. "If that nurse had been in my bloody shoes," I told myself, "I bet she would have made damn sure that she had a relaxant before facing any form surgery." Now you know why I emphasised earlier the importance of ensuring that you clearly inform those dealing with your case that you want pre-med drugs.

I remember thinking also how, in this day and age, some nurses just seemed uninterested in the job that they do. Being the patient, I wanted to feel there was someone there to help me get through my ordeal; on this occasion that had not been the case.

I looked in the direction of the frail old lady opposite me, wondering again what might have happened if I had not bothered to help her. Would she have had no breakfast? Would the staff have assumed that she was not hungry and therefore her tray would have been removed? I tortured myself with those thoughts.

Slowly, I pulled the curtains around my bed, removed my own clothes and put on the theatre gown. I did not open the curtains when ready. I honestly don't think I could have spoken to anyone at that time as I was so very close to openly crying. Cap in hand, I just sat there in my own little world. What else could I do? I had no power or say in the decision of whether or not I should have a pre-med, nor did I have control of my life; it was now once again in other people's hands.

Soon after, a junior nurse popped her head through the curtain to make sure I was alright and to let me know that she would be escorting me to theatre. She told me that she would also be joining me in the operating theatre to watch my surgery. I couldn't believe my ears; I wasn't very happy. Who did she think she was, assuming she had the right to attend without even having the decency to ask me if I minded? "No bloody way," I thought, as anger consumed me. I might have been the type of person that would be obliging and support trainee nurses in their quest to learn, but not this time. No one considered my feelings on the subject. I just was not having it and I was going to make damn sure that on this I got my own way.

Not long afterwards, I was once again being wheeled down the corridors on my way to the operating theatre, junior nurse in tow. Once there, as before, my details were checked and double-checked by two theatre nurses and Little Miss High and Mighty. As this was being done, the student nurse spoke above the others, informing them that her ward sister had said that she could stay to watch my surgery. I instantly shot a discontented glance at one of the theatre nurses, letting her know that I was not happy about the arrangement.

On seeing my reaction, the theatre nurse automatically replied, "No, that will not be possible; requests to join the theatre team must be made prior to the day of surgery."

With that, she then returned to checking my paperwork. The junior nurse was left speechless and rather embarrassed. She sheepishly stood in silence until all my formalities were completed and then went on her way back to the ward, with not even a goodbye. As I looked at the theatre nurse, I remember thinking that this was certainly someone who was a real nurse, someone who took the time to consider how I felt and then professionally dealt with the situation. I thanked her for her understanding.

Not long after that, I was being asked to transfer from the trolley onto one of the theatre beds and then once again lined up with the rest of the beds that lay side by side in what you could call a holding bay, whilst I waited to be taken to theatre.

As I lay there, I noticed that this time I was not on my own; there was another woman lying about two beds from me who, like myself, was obviously also going in for surgery. Eyes closed, it seemed apparent to me that she had been fortunate and had received a pre-med, because she seemed relaxed and unaware that I had come into the room.

My nerves engulfed me and I found I had an overwhelming urge at that point to get up out of the bed and walk away. I just wanted to scream. I was not coping with the situation that I found myself in at all; it was as if I almost wanted to put up my hand and say, "Alright cancer, you win; I can't take anymore."

Trying so desperately to control my emotions, I told myself, "You can do this Roseann." I could cry when I recall these feelings. Taking deep breaths, I tried desperately to calm myself down. Thoughts of my family shot through my mind. I really believe that had not been for them, I would have given up.

Once in the operating theatre, a comforting male voice behind me was instructing me to breathe deeply into the mask that now surrounded my nose and mouth. By this time I was so emotionally drained that I almost felt relieved in knowing that I would soon be unconscious and temporarily free from this nightmare.

Waking in recovery, my consciousness was momentary. I remember opening my eyes and that was it. I didn't remember much else about my time spent there and was surprised to find that I was back in my bed within the ward the next time I opened my eyes.

Most of the day I drifted in and out of consciousness. When I did eventually start to become more like myself, I was surprised to find it was early evening. Instantly I was aware that I had more movement in my left arm; it was almost as if someone had cut an invisible string, one that had been preventing my arm from moving in a normal fashion. I remember thinking to myself that maybe my mother would get off my back. I felt relief in the knowledge that when I told people I was unable to move my arm, I wasn't going mad.

When I apprehensively lifted the hospital gown away from my body to look at my chest, all I could see were large mounds of dressing that covered a now very flat area where my breast had once been. I could also see two tubes protruding from the dressing and knew on inspecting them more closely that they were drainage tubes.

Physically, I felt as though I had been assaulted. I was very sore around my wound area and extremely uncomfortable. When I tried to move even slightly, I experienced problems. I found it impossible to sit up unaided and that scared me; I had no strength. I was now also experiencing a sensation of extreme tightness around my body, almost as if my skin had been stretched to its limit.

Later, I did manage to freshen up with the help of a nurse. After washing and changing my nightdress, I did feel slightly better, but only briefly. This time around, I definitely felt a lot worse.

Visiting time arrived and although not feeling that great, I was excited at the prospect of seeing John. I watched him closely as he walked in the direction of my bed, overcome with love for him. He had been there for me, right by my side, ready to do anything without a moan or a groan.

I told him about everything that had happened with regard to the pre-med and how the young nurse had assumed she could just waltz in on my surgery, but none of that really mattered now as I focused on the fact that my arm had returned to what I assumed as normal. John looked so pleased when he heard that part of my news.

Tiredness overwhelmed me quickly during John's visit and I found myself struggling to stay awake. On occasions I would only realise that I had actually nodded off when I would startle myself back to reality, which inevitably made John laugh. At the end of visiting time, I kissed John goodnight and literally slumped back onto the pillows on my bed, grateful for the fact that I could once again sleep.

I felt so sore; the area around my wound felt extremely tight and was throbbing like hell. As one of the nurses passed, I called out to her and asked if she could get me something for my pain. I tried to turn myself onto my side to see if changing position would provide some relief, but I found it too painful even to do that. Instead, I opted for remaining in my current position until the nurse returned and administered my much needed pain relief. I fell asleep shortly afterwards and with the exception of the odd time when I did wake up and flinch with pain, my night was uneventful.

When I awoke next morning at around 5.30am, my body felt as though it had permanently seized up and my pain appeared to be worse. I felt relieved at being able to catch the attention of one of night nurses as she walked by.

"Could you give me something for my pain?" I whispered.

As the nurse began to administer morphine into a small tube with a cap on the end of it, I felt almost instant relief. I remember being amazed on the very first occasion it was used; it was a little contraption that protruded from a vein in my neck. I presumed it had been put in place whilst I was in theatre. No stingy injections for me this time around.

"How are you coping? You have certainly been through the mill," the nurse said, as she sat herself on the edge of my bed.

I think I must have released every fear, worry and discomfort I had experienced since being diagnosed with breast cancer to this woman. It was such a comfort having someone to talk to that for once I could say exactly how I felt. I could cry in front of her, be myself and tell her all my fears, all without having to worry about upsetting her. She was a true professional who most probably heard similar stories to mine on a weekly basis and had most probably learned to detach herself to a certain degree to prevent herself from getting too involved, but even if that were in case, she showed true understanding and compassion to my situation.

With my family and friends, I could not do that. I didn't want to cause them more pain or make them cry, something I would have done if I had shared with them the feelings and fears that were deep within me. I already knew they were hurting badly because of my illness; how could I add to that?

It was truly amazing having someone there for me. That nurse really helped me that morning just by taking the time to listen. Even now the impact of her actions still prove to me that there are nurses out there that do make a great difference in our lives and I try so very hard to remember that. God bless her.

After pouring out my heart to the nurse, I dozed on and off up until breakfast time. With the assistance of one of the male nurses, I managed to get myself into an upright position at the side of my bed.

I didn't much feel like eating and in fact would have been happy with just a hot mug of tea. However, I knew that the tea now given in national health hospitals comes from a machine and is absolutely disgusting, not to mention cold by the time you get it. Instead, I opted for a glass of my juice from a bottle that John had bought me the day before, whilst I pondered on how the hell I was going to manage a shower.

The male nurse returned, this time to inform me that at some point in the morning my dressings would be removed and my wound re-dressed. He then told me that he would be the person that would be doing the procedure. I felt immediate panic. There was no way I could let this male nurse look at my body; it was just too unthinkable. How could he honestly think that I would not be horrified by what he was suggesting? It was bad enough having to face up to the fact that I had just lost a very important and intimate part of my body, without also having to go through the indignity of having to expose this area to a person of the oppose sex. I just couldn't.

I know some of you out there might say to yourself that he was a nurse and was used to it, but try to put yourself in my position. Here I was, being told by a man 15 years younger than I that he would be the one by my side when my dressings were being removed for the first time. This was a situation that required both sensitivity and understanding. He could not understand how the removal of a breast had affected me, or how it now made me feel less of a woman. He would also be unable to understand how degraded I would feel when he looked at my body.

Once I had calmed myself down, I asked to speak to the sister of the ward. On explaining to her how I felt, she instantly understood and reassuringly she told me that she would come back later and do my dressing personally. I felt so relieved.

When I told the male nurse that I had expressed my wishes to the sister, he appeared peeved. However, it didn't bother me, because his temporary moment of upset was nothing compared to how I would have felt if helped by him. Ironically, neither the male nurse nor the ward sister did the procedure, as not long after my surgeon Alison arrived. After having a quick peek behind my dressing, she told me that my wound appeared weepy. She asked Jean to get her an iodine dressing. "This will dry up your wound," she told me as she applied it.

During Alison's visit, I told her of the terrible tightness that I was experiencing around my chest area and asked if anything could be done to ease it. She told me that she had expected me to have this problem, then went on to tell me that this was because I had very little skin left around my surgery site.

"You should have seen the trouble I had trying to make the ends meet," she said jokingly. "It will ease off through time," she then said reassuringly.

As our conversation continued, the subject of chemotherapy came up. My ears went up like a shot as I looked directly into my surgeon's face, now with warning bells once again ringing in my ears.

"Some patients' post op treatment does include a course of chemotherapy," Alison told me.

I found it hard to take in her words. I could feel the familiar sense of panic rise within me as well as confusion. Chemotherapy had never been mentioned before in any of my consultations with Alison; even the word made me feel physically sick.

I had always had a very open and honest relationship with the doctors and nurses that had been involved in my care, but that did not mean that being hit with the prospect of having to go through chemotherapy was any easier. I felt as if every time

I relaxed and let my guard down in the slightest, believing that things were beginning to go my way, something else would happen that would force me right back to the bottom of the hill I was so desperately trying to climb. I was beginning to wonder just how many more knocks I could take.

Jean tried to take the edge off the tension that had now filled the small area around my bed, telling me of how great advances had been made and how this form of treatment was nothing like people perceived it to be. Nevertheless, her words made me feel no better.

Knowing me as she did, Jean also knew that I would want to know as much about my impending treatment as possible.

"I will come back later, most probably this afternoon, with some fact sheets. Then you will be able to get a better insight and understanding of what it entails."

I sat in silence once Jean and Alison had left, trying so very hard to make sense of what I had just been told. Did that mean that my cancer had been worse than they anticipated? Was I doomed to die and the chemotherapy treatment was only really being given in the hope that it would give me more time? These were just a couple of the morbid thoughts that invaded my mind, in addition to all the horror stories I had heard with regard to this form of treatment.

A nurse was now by my side and I wasn't even aware that she had approached me. She asked if I was alright. Obviously Jean had spoken to her and told her of my reaction to the news. Most probably knowing Jean, she had asked the nurse if she would keep an eye on me. That was the kind of person she was; kind, understanding and thoughtful.

Tears began to run down my face as I tried hard to tell the nurse that I would be alright. However, she knew otherwise and automatically began drawing the curtains around my bed to give me some privacy. The nurse and I spoke for a short time. Again, I was so very grateful for her support and reassurance and eventually I calmed down, although I remained absolutely devastated by the news.

The remainder of that morning was hell. I wondered how John and I were going to manage to continue paying our mortgage. There was no way I would be returning to work in the near future and I would soon be running out of sick pay. All the horror stories of chemotherapy were also plaguing my mind, as were thoughts of how I would cope with losing my hair. No sooner had I calmed myself down, than the words mortgage, chemotherapy and baldness would flash through my mind and I would be off again in floods of tears.

John had told me the night before that my sister-in law had planned to visit me that afternoon during her lunch hour. I also knew that my mother would be up to visit as well. I told myself I would have to buck up or I would not be in any fit state to see my mother. It was this that gave me strength, for I knew my poor mum would be devastated. I needed to be strong for her. I lay on top of my bed and tried to clear all negative thoughts from my mind.

I hadn't been able to muster up an appetite, so declined lunch, but did opt to take a cup of horrible hospital tea; how I would have loved a decent cup. For the remainder of the time leading up to visiting hour, I lay on top of my bed and stared into space, with the exception of the time that it took me to shower. I hadn't experienced much pain that day and was at least glad of that. I don't think I could have coped with everything that had happened that day as well as pain. Whether or not it was the adrenalin now pumping around my body that kept my pain at bay I don't know, but I was grateful for the respite.

Cancer No Not Me!

I had noticed that there was a chair positioned at the end of the corridor that faced directly up the ward. On pulling a pillow from my bed, I shuffled towards it slowly, then eased myself into it. Getting down into the chair was a struggle but worth it, for once seated I was amazed at how comfortable I felt. I just watched everyone, from nurses to patients, going back and forth, relieved that by doing so, my mind was temporarily clear of gloomy thoughts.

Jean did return as she said she would. Automatically, she helped me out of the chair, then walked with me to my bed. Drawing the curtains, we both sat on the edge of my bed. Jean spoke first.

"I have fact sheets for you on a few chemotherapy treatments and also a booklet on a drug called Tamoxifen."

"More treatment," I remember thinking to myself.

I couldn't believe this was happening.

"What is Tamoxifen?" I asked Jean.

"It is a drug that is widely used and prescribed to people who have been diagnosed with breast cancer. It is known to reduce the chances of reoccurrence. You knew you would require some form of treatment."

"Yes," I said, "but never for I minute did I expect to be told that I needed chemotherapy. I was just coming to terms with the fact that I might have had to go through radiotherapy treatment and now I'm being told that I may require both, plus ongoing drug therapy."

Lying on my bed after Jean had left, I lifted the fact sheet on chemotherapy and began to read: "Chemotherapy: – Frequently asked questions". It covered many different issues and explained things such as the importance of informing the doctors of any other drugs you are taking, or additional drugs you would like to take; this even included things like vitamins, something that you would have thought was not worth mentioning. It told you of the possibilities of planning your treatment around a vacation, but with regard to going abroad they advised against it. Organisations were also highlighted where you could receive helpful advice. Further on, it mentioned that being told that chemotherapy is part of your recommended treatment can evoke a range of emotions. They say that some people feel positive and secure in the knowledge that everything possible is being done for them. Others can feel much like I did; anxious and frightened. It also said that this is sometimes due to the person mistakenly believing that chemotherapy is only given when the cancer has spread, or is more serious; thoughts that had crossed my mind.

The fact sheet stated that these days chemotherapy is commonly given even when there is no evidence of spread and in addition to surgery and/or radiotherapy as a form of "insurance policy". It all made good sense, but didn't really appease me. It's all good reading when it isn't happening to you personally.

I turned to the booklet headed "Tamoxifen", anxious to read what it had to say. It told of how Tamoxifen was a hormonal drug commonly used as part of the treatment for breast cancer. It is also described as an anti-oestrogen drug. Apparently, it is thought to work in several ways although at present all its actions are not completely known.

It told of how some breast cancers are stimulated by the female hormone oestrogen, which encourages cells to grow. These cancers are known as oestrogen receptor positive tumours. Tamoxifen works by blocking the effects of oestrogen on cancer cells, so stopping them from growing. Some breast cancers that are oestrogen receptor negative may also sometimes respond to Tamoxifen; however, the benefits are greater when the tumour is oestrogen receptor positive. It also told of how this drug had, as Jean said, been shown to decrease the chances of tumour recurrence and that it apparently improved the chances of survival following surgery for breast cancer, as well as reducing the risk of cancer in the other breast by 38%. Listing its side effects, it highlighted that these are greatest in pre-menopausal patients, but very rarely is it required for the drug to be stopped.

Mild indigestion, nausea, hot flushes and vaginal discharge or dryness are all noted side effects and in some people they experience lighter periods by 25% and in others, they stop altogether (50%). Hair and nail growth may slow down and hair may become coarser. Some people also may put on weight.

Everything that I had read with regard to any forthcoming treatments I required seemed a bit like swings and roundabouts. In other words, some treatments may help you in one way, but at the same time may cause problems in other areas. However, I drew the conclusion that when it came down to hard facts, I would try anything in my fight to stay alive.

My sister-in law Maggie was walking in my direction, smiling as I caught her attention. Once she had sat down, I told her how it had been explained to me that I may require chemotherapy. The look on her face told me how shocked she was at hearing my news. "Don't worry. I'm fine about it," I lied.

On then trying to tell her how I felt when I thought about the words mortgage, chemotherapy and baldness, my emotions engulfed me and I was unable to say anymore. Quickly I grabbed for a tissue to dry my eyes, unable to tell her just how much these words affected me.

I had managed to regain my composure and within minutes my mother had arrived. Perplexed, I looked to see who had come with her.

"Debbie is trying to find a parking space; I could wait no longer to see you, so I got her to drop me off and came right up," my mum explained as she took a seat.

Debbie was my youngest sister. I took a deep breath and tried with all my might to be strong.

"Mum, they told me today that I may need chemotherapy. Now I don't want you worrying about it because I am fine. I was just telling Maggie that it is only when I think of three words, mortgage, chemotherapy and baldness … ." It had happened again; I had lost control and began crying again.

This was truly one of the hardest things I had ever had to do through all of this and it broke my heart. There I was openly crying my eyes out in front of my poor mother. I had wanted to be strong for her; I could not bear to see her upset. It was just too painful. On seeing my tears, my mother instantly began to cry also. That had been the last thing that I had wanted to happen. Rising from the edge of my bed, I cupped my mother's face in my hands, telling her between sobs that everything was going to be alright. I felt so helpless. I wanted so much to take away my mother's pain, but could not. She was tearing apart inside and I could do nothing.

One of the nurses entered the hospital bay and sympathetically she put her arm around my mother and reassured her whilst walking her towards the nursing station. With my sister-in-law by my side, I tried to recompose myself before my mother's return.

I was so thankful that my youngest sister had not been there to experience the emotional breakdown of my mother and me, for I truly believe she too would have fallen apart.

Shortly after my mother returned with the nurse by her side.

"Are you alright?" the nurse asked me.

Telling her I was, I thanked her for looking after my mother.

My young sister did not appear until halfway through the visiting hour, rather exasperated due to the problems she had experienced in finding a parking space. She was totally oblivious to what had taken place earlier. This time as I told her how I may require chemotherapy treatment, I made sure that I did not repeat the words that had caused me to become so upset.

By around 5.30pm, the pain I experienced at my wound site was intense. Lying on my bed, I tried hard to focus on things that were important to me. I thought of my grandchildren and their short lives to date, going over in my head all the good things we had done together since they had come into this world. I also envisaged what the future held, hoping that I would still be alive to see them mature into young women. I thought about my mum and dad, recalling funny and happy times that had taken place as I was growing up. I also promised myself that I would spend more time with them, well aware now of how quickly our lives can change.

Thoughts of my sisters made me laugh away to myself as I remembered silly little incidents from the past; like the time when I was 12-years-old and my mother and father had gone out for the evening, leaving my oldest sister Issy to watch over the rest of us. As soon as our parents had left the house, Issy instantly warned us that we had better behave, as she walked into her bedroom to get away from us. My younger sister Janet had long flowing hair and at that time, the pageboy hair cut was the "in" thing. Through suggestion and continual coaxing, she had agreed that I could cut her hair in that same style. I had always wanted to be a hairdresser, you see, and thought this was my ideal opportunity to show my talent.

As I cut away at my sister's lovely long hair, I found that I just couldn't get the sides the same, so I then would cut a bit more, then another bit more. Before I knew it, my poor little sister's hair was up at her ears. I thought it hysterical now as I had a picture of her in my head sitting on that chair with most of her hair on the floor, with a style more like a bowl cut than a pageboy.

Given that there were five of us, we were always moaning or arguing with each other. I would often hear my mother's voice yet again telling us that it was terrible that we constantly bickered with each other, adding, "I don't understand you girls. When I was growing up, I never argued with my sister; I was just grateful that I had one".

Memories of my son Billy growing up flashed through my mind. When he was only 3-years-old he had this blue and white woolly hat that he just adored. He would wear it everywhere he went; even to bed. I would have to wait every night until he had fallen asleep before I could remove it from his head. When I did, there would be beads of sweat all over his forehead. He looked so cute and angelic lying there fast asleep.

I recalled how when John and I first met we didn't really like each other and usually tried to avoid each other like the plague. However, that was difficult due to the fact that we had the same circle of friends. But strangely enough, as we got to know each other better, we grew closer and closer. That was 12 years previously. Now he was my darling husband, who I must say, I wouldn't swap for the world. I felt truly blessed by the life I had and knew how very lucky I was to have such a wonderful family.

My pain, however, remained and as I saw the ward sister go by I called to her and asked if she could give me something to relieve it. On telling me she would, I rested my head back onto my pillow and waited for her to return. Some time had passed and I was beginning to wonder just where the ward sister had gone; she had obviously had other things she needed to do and I was well aware of that, but wished she would come and give me something for my steadily increasing pain. I told myself that I would wait a little longer and when either the sister or one of the nurses passed, I would again ask for pain relief. I hated pressing those bells that are situated by your bed; I always imagine that when a patient presses one of them, it only irritates the nurses if they are in the middle of doing something else.

I think my experiences of the day had also helped to knock my own pain threshold out of sync, first by numbing it and then by increasing it to a higher pitch than I had ever experienced. It was either that or I had exceeded the time when my medication should have been due and the last dose had worn off.

I remember pleading in my mind for someone to come and administer some morphine, but again I waited. By this time my pain was so bad that it brought tears to my eyes. I just felt so very low and was beginning to believe that no one on the ward cared, or was interested in how I felt. Of course, I know that I most probably felt like that because of my increasing inability to cope with my pain and the emotions that it had triggered.

My Godsend turned out to be not far away; the ward domestic assistant. On seeing how distressed I had become,

Cancer No Not Me!

she took it upon herself to go and fetch the ward sister. Words can't express how grateful I was at this girl's compassion and kindness. Shortly afterwards, I was given my morphine and my pain was once again at bay.

John and our son Billy were amazingly supportive to me when they visited that evening, trying their best for my sake to remain calm and lighthearted. At one point we were all actually laughing at the thought of me with a bald head. John and Billy told me that when that time came, they would also shave their heads, then we would all look the same. They certainly managed to make feel more like my old self again. They also made me believe that with them beside me I could beat this awful disease. I loved them both so very much.

Visiting hour seemed to go so fast that evening and when the bell rang to let relatives know that it was time for them to go, I could almost feel a blanket of blackness wash over me as tears fill my eyes once more. I did not want to be there; I wanted to be home with my family. On seeing me become upset John said, "Don't worry; it won't be long 'til you're back home". He also joked that he was enjoying the rest, by continuing, "God woman, give me a chance to recharge my batteries so that I am able to look after you when you do come home". I knew that he was only saying this to try and pep my spirits up. I smiled at him, telling him that I would be alright. Billy kissed me goodbye, telling me that he would go so that John and I could have a few minutes by ourselves, ending with, "I will be back to see you tomorrow. Love you".

In the few minutes that were left of the visiting hour, John and I kissed and said our goodbyes.

"Phone me later if you can manage," he told me, as I watched him walk away.

Cancer No Not Me!

Throughout the rest of that night I gradually became more and more downhearted. The events of the day had now gripped hold of me and all I could think about was when I was going to die. The longer I was alone, the more the thoughts of survival diminished. I did try to mix with the other patients that shared the hospital bay, but it was so very hard. I was the only one that had been admitted for cancer surgery, so therefore found no common ground between myself and the three other women.

The older woman that I had helped with breakfast on my first morning in hospital was very confused and spent most of the time looking into space, appearing to be caught up in her own thoughts. One of the other women I had spoken to briefly told me how I had been totally out of it when I had returned from theatre. "All you did when you got back was continually open and shut your eyes and at afternoon visiting when your eyes were opened, you would stare blankly at my visitors," she had said. Afterwards she had told me that she had been admitted for some stomach problems and had been in for almost a week.

The remaining patient had an array of health problems and told me how she had spent a good part of her life in hospital. So there we were; a true mixture of sick people, all thrown together in one bay.

My mood did not lift as I telephoned our house to speak to John later that evening. On hearing his voice, I instantly began to cry. Through tears I blurted out all my fears and admitted how I could not stop thinking that I would not have long on this earth. I had really got myself into a state at one point during our conversation, for John kept insisting that I go and speak to a nurse. "Tell them how upset you are." But I didn't want to; I did not want them to know how poorly I was coping.

John must have felt so helpless at the other end of that phone, knowing how distressed I was and being unable to do anything about it. I always feel guilty about what I put him through that night, even though he tells me that's what he was there for; a shoulder to cry on. Through constant reassurance, jokes and tender loving words, John eventually managed to calm me down and by the end of our telephone conversation my tears had dried up. I returned to my bed after that and waited for my nightly medication, hoping that it would not be long before I fell asleep and put an end to my truly horrible day.

On one of the mornings that Jean had popped in to see me, she told me that three woman had been admitted the previous night, all of whom were scheduled to have breast cancer surgery. "They are all in a bay together at the top of the ward," she said. Not going into any of the three women's personal details, she told me how anxious they all appeared. "Maybe if they had the chance to speak to someone like yourself that has already gone through the surgery, it may help them," she suggested.

She didn't have to say another word. I knew exactly what she meant. Jean knew that I would try my best to reassure them as well as attempt to ease any fears they might have had, whilst they waited to go to theatre. I felt fulfilled when helping others and even if I could take away or reduce the anxiety in the smallest way of even one of these women, then I would have felt like the person I once was for the first time since being diagnosed.

I brushed my hair and even put on a bit of mascara and blusher. I wanted to show these women that what they were about to experience was not the end of the world. Slowly,

Cancer No Not Me!

I made my way to the other end of the ward. Walking into the bay alone made me feel sad, as I was instantly faced with such a tense atmosphere and a cloud of gloom. I found myself wondering whether I looked the same as these women now did the first time I took that journey to theatre and into the unknown. Looking at them, I wanted so much to take away their anxieties, something that I know was impossible for they too had to face this journey on their own. I could only attempt to offer some momentary relief.

As I spoke to these women, I thanked God that my surgery was now behind me. Obviously, these were thoughts that I would have never shared with them. As Jean had said, they were all feeling very low. Introducing myself, I tried to appear upbeat but relaxed. I then took a seat and began a conversation. I told of how this had been my second surgery, making sure though that I highlighted that no two people were alike. I didn't want to heighten their fears by giving them dreaded thoughts that they too could find themselves in similar circumstances to mine. I wanted, if anything, to instil thoughts of "Well at least we're not as bad as she is".

I was amazed by how our conversation developed and of how open we instantly became with one another. One told me she had a young daughter and of how so many of her female relations had all been diagnosed in the past with breast cancer. "It's hereditary," she explained. She then went on to tell me that because so many in her family had been diagnosed with this awful disease, doctors were now looking into her family background to see whether or not there was a gene that could be responsible. It was hoped that by testing her daughter, they would be able to determine if she would be at risk of developing breast cancer when she was older. She was only about ten, I think. I remember thinking to myself, "And

I was trying to heighten confidence in this woman." After speaking to her, I began to think that I was the lucky one. It's a true saying: "There is always someone out there worse off than you", something I could now clearly see.

Another of the women was much older than the rest of us; she appeared to be in her sixties. She seemed to be coping a lot better than the other two, commenting on how thankful she was at seeing me and how it had helped to ease her nerves a bit. If the truth be told, she seemed more concerned about the third woman. In a whisper, she began to tell me that this woman and her daughters were having great difficulty in accepting her diagnosis. On speaking with this woman myself, I could identify with her emotions, as they were almost the mirror image of mine, except that I did not openly discuss them. She was at the stage that I knew only too well, believing that she would not get better and thinking only of death. I tried so very hard to reassure her as much as possible.

As our surgeon Alison entered the room with Jean at her side, she jokingly said, "So I see you've met trouble", obviously meaning me. I did not stay much longer, for I knew that she had come to speak to each of them about their forthcoming surgery. As I slowly walked back to my bed, I felt a great feeling of satisfaction at knowing that I had been there for these women, something I wished I had experienced when I first needed surgery for my breast cancer.

When I had returned to my bed, I mulled over my encounter with these women. The more I thought about how Jean had highlighted their presence, the more I began to realise that it was not only for the benefit of these women, but was also for mine. Jean knew that she would trigger the desire in me to help others, given that she also knew that by giving me an objective, she would boost my confidence and self-esteem, not to mention help me to face my own fears.

I only hope I helped that day.

Whilst in hospital this time around, I had a most unpleasant experience of meeting a nurse with a poor bedside manner who, when giving out the daily medication, made you feel as if you almost had to beg for pain killing drugs. She was really a very intimidating individual who I am sure would have brought anyone feeling really low to tears. I know that on my first encounter with her, I felt rather awkward, almost to the point of feeling like a small child. It wasn't until I had actually pondered over what had happened when first we met, that I became angry with myself for letting this person make me feel that way. You would have truly thought by the way in which she reacted that she personally owned the medication that she administered.

On a few occasions, I had noted her response when I had asked her for a stronger painkiller after she handed me two paracetamol. She would instantly draw me a look that said, "Oh you don't really need that". I remember thinking to myself, "Well if you were to step into my body for a short while, then maybe you'd understand why I do."

Now given that I had become stronger within myself, I could handle the situation. I spoke to Jean, asking if she would emphasise to the nursing staff the importance of these drugs in my treatment. After all, I had enough to cope with and didn't need unnecessary pain on top of everything else.

The point that I am trying to make is the huge difference a little thing like a stronger painkiller, for instance, can aid someone's recovery. Pain is a terrible thing; it makes you irritable and causes you to experience difficulty when trying to concentrate on even the simplest of tasks. It also inevitably causes the soapy bubbles (tears). If you are the patient, it's your body, so don't doubt the pain you feel; it is real. Don't "make do", because it will only be harder on you in the long run.

As for those of you who are family members and friends of a cancer sufferer, try not to take it to heart when your loved one bites your head off for no apparent reason, because it is not you personally that we mean to hurt; sometimes we just can't help ourselves and we do truly feel remorseful for upsetting you.

The removal of my drains is an important topic that should not be overlooked. I feel it would be a beneficial subject of discussion that may help to alleviate fears of the unknown and also help those facing surgery to obtain a better understanding about something that may be alien to them, or causing them some concern.

As I had mentioned earlier, I did in fact have two drains inserted at different sites of my wound, which were held in position by a few small stitches. The drains themselves are positioned whilst you are in the operating theatre when you are anaesthetised. You will be relieved to know you are totally unaware of the procedure taking place. The tube from each drain is connected to a small, balloon like plastic ball, which works, I believe, as a way of suctioning out any excess blood or foreign matter from the wound site. All fluid gradually flows from the tube into a small disposable bag at the end of the drain tubing. Nursing staff are then able to determine when your drains should be removed, based on the amount of fluid that passes from them.

I know that it all sounds rather gruesome, but it is an ingenious piece of equipment that performs a very important job and really isn't that unsightly. My drains caused slight discomfort and, on a few occasions, felt as if they had nipped me slightly internally when I would turn too quickly, or when I would lie in a certain position, but personally the discomfort in my opinion was minimal. They were more of a nuisance than anything.

When being removed, a nurse will snip the stitches that hold the drain in position. He or she will then tell you to take a deep breath, explaining that as the drain is being removed you should give a long breath out, no stopping in the middle. The reason for this is, I think, a way of distracting your attention from the drain by redirecting all your concentration to that of breathing as instructed. As it is removed, you experience a rather strange sensation, almost like the sensation you feel when you remove a hair from your mouth, but on a larger scale. It is slightly uncomfortable, but in my experience not painful and is over in a matter of seconds. After your drains have been removed, the feeling of freedom you experience is fantastic. You also no longer have the performance of having to constantly carry them around.

A funny part of having a drain or drains is that when you are able to walk about, one of the nursing staff proudly hands you a plastic shopping bag to carry them around in. I could not stop laughing when this happened to me.

On another of the days whilst still in hospital, Jean came to visit me carrying with her an attractive looking bag. Intrigued, I just had to ask her what it contained. To my surprise, the bag contained a breast prosthesis, something to which I had not even given a thought, let alone wanted to see, but that did not stop her from showing me anyway. She explained how the prosthesis was one known as a "softy". This was, she said, because it was filled with a very soft cotton

Cancer No Not Me!

wool like substance. "It's ideal for you at the moment, given that your body is still in the process of healing," she told me.

Jean had such a bubbly personality, an ideal person for the job that she did; a true professional in every sense of the word. Trying her best to create an atmosphere of excitement, she happily presented the prosthesis to me as if handing me a present. "Look," she said, "you can fill it to the size that matches your own breast," she enthused. I had to admit she was certainly trying her best to make a very sensitive subject pleasant. She did not push the issue or make a comment of how once worn it looked like the real thing to the outside world. Instead, she highlighted how, by slipping it snugly into my bra, it just might help to restore some of my confidence lost with the removal of my breast. After Jean had left, I put the bag containing my new left breast at the side of my bed. I wasn't quite ready to rush into the world of prostheses. I needed time.

Later that day, after much thought, I then selected a bra and took it, along with the carrier bag containing the false breast, towards the toilet. If I was going to try it on, it needed to be when I was alone and behind a locked door. I did not want to be taking my first steps trying out a prosthesis, only to find a nurse popping their head through curtains I had drawn around my bed. If something like that were to happen, I think I would have just wanted to curl up and die. I had to maintain my dignity.

Behind the locked door of the bathroom, alone and happy that no one could walk in on me, I then slowly removed the false breast from its box. Gently, I fastened my bra and looking full frontal into the mirror, I gently slipped the prosthesis into the space that my left breast had once filled. Pulling down one of my very baggy t-shirts that I now wore,

I looked directly into the mirror once again, pleasantly surprised at the image of how I once was reflecting back at me. I was happy that for the first time since my surgery I felt like a woman again.

From then on, I knew there was no looking back. The false breast might not have been perfect, but to those who were unaware of the fact that I had lost my left breast, I looked no different from any other woman and that is how I needed to feel.

During one of the conversations I had with Jean, I asked her what my actual chance of survival was, explaining to her that this was something I needed to know. I know that a lot of people choose not to be told the finer details of their medical outcomes, but I needed to know for many reasons. I am the type of person that has to know what they are up against in order to gain the strength to fight. Another reason for feeling as I did was that a work colleague of mine had died suddenly only a short while after returning home from work one evening. It had horrified me to think that here was this poor woman who had spent her last few precious hours working. I felt so sorry that she had not been given the chance to share those hours with the people she loved. Feeling as I did about this, I had always promised myself that if ever I were told that I was seriously ill, then I would make damn sure that every living moment that I had left would be spent with the people that I loved.

If my prognosis was not favourable, then there were things I felt I had to address. I wanted to have the time to reinforce the love I had to all the people that were important in my life. I wanted to be able to do as many of the things that I had dreamt of doing that I had put on the back burner due to lack of money, or because I just never took the time. Sadly, I knew that the unspoken subject of a funeral would eventually arise and have to be addressed. I know it may sound mad or morbid, but these are truly all the things that run through your mind when you think that you are going to die. The realisation that you might possibly only have a very short time sends you into a state of panic.

Expressing all these feelings to Jean, she understood and respected how I felt.

"At your next appointment with Alison, tell her how you feel," Jean advised.

I made up my mind to do just that.

Chapter Eight

Will I Ever Get Out of Here?

The morning of my discharge had arrived and after showering I eagerly sought out the ward sister to ask how soon I could go home. However, disappointment instantly set in when she informed me that she was unable to tell me there and then.

"I have to first speak to the medical team who are dealing with your case. As soon as I hear anything I will let you know."

I felt so frustrated at having to wait, as it was only around 8.30am and I knew that it would be well into the morning before the doctors did their rounds. In an attempt to pacify myself, I bought a daily paper from the trolley stand that came to the ward on a daily basis. However, I could not concentrate; I was too excited at the prospect of going home.

I must have walked around the ward at least five times that morning as I tried to pass time. At around 10.30am Jean popped in to see how I was getting on. Telling her I was fine, I then eagerly asked her if she would be able to find out any information on when I would be discharged. I didn't see the point of sitting about all morning only to be told some hours later that the doctor had said it was alright for me to go via a telephone conversation. Jean told me that she would try her best and would get back to me when she had more information. More waiting.

It was another hour before Jean eventually got back to me. I waited for her to speak, ready to hang onto her every word and hoping all the while that she would say I was free to go. No such luck; she informed me that it was preferred that I wait until 2pm.

"Why?" I asked in a rather irked manner.

"The doctors involved in your case want to see you at the combined breast cancer clinic before they confirm that it is alright for you to go home," Jean explained.

I telephoned John for what must have been about the fourth time that morning, telling him of how peeved I was at the thought of having to mull around the ward until the clinic had started.

"Calm yourself; it won't be long now," he reassured me.

All my belongings sat there neatly packed and ready to go. I felt like just picking them up and walking out the door, but I knew I couldn't. Lying on top of my bed, I had an instant brain wave. What if I told John to come up a few hours before the start of the clinic? We could then at least go for lunch together. I only hoped that the ward sister would agree to me having my lunch in the hospital canteen rather than in the ward. Excitedly, I went in search of her. I was over the moon when she said she had no problem in allowing me to leave the ward. However, she did make me promise that I would not leave the hospital until after I had been seen at the clinic. I made my way once again to the telephone, happy that I would soon be able to leave the ward at least.

After telling John my bright idea, I then asked him to come up as soon as he could. I was more content now; the time I had to wait for John to arrive was nothing, knowing that I would soon be able to roam around the hospital. That would definitely help the time to go quickly.

It was a great feeling when I eventually walked from the ward and into the hospital corridors, with only the formality of being discharged via the clinic. I was free and I felt invigorated after being in hospital for five days. I couldn't wait to get back to normality.

Funnily enough, I wasn't even hungry, but that did not matter; I would be quite content sitting sipping tea and watching the world go by as I waited for the time of my clinic appointment to arrive.

Later, as we entered the clinic area, I wasn't surprised to see it overflowing with people as usual. I informed the receptionist that I had just come from the ward and it had been arranged that I see the breast team at the clinic. I then took a seat and waited for my name to be called.

I must admit that by that time I didn't feel that grand; exhaustion had quickly washed over me and I felt totally drained. The pain had also begun to creep back once more. I remember commenting to John that it was strange how you seem to feel ten times worse once you have left a ward environment.

I was surprised when an hour had passed and I still hadn't been seen. I thought that given that I had just been through major surgery and the fact that I had come via a ward, someone would have considered these factors and would have made a point of seeing me sooner rather than later, but that was not the case. The more time passed by, the more distressed I became at not being able to go home. I seriously needed to lie down. Every muscle and bone in my body ached the longer I sat on the hard plastic chairs in the waiting area. John had wanted to go over to the receptionist on a few occasions to enquire why the doctors were taking so long to see me, but I persuaded him not to, hoping that I would be called at any time. However, after another hour had passed with no sign of being seen, I then relented, finding myself now almost pleading with John to speak to the receptionist and emphasise the problems that I was experiencing.

The receptionist got to her feet and walked into the area of the clinic that contained the consultation rooms after John had spoken to her.

"What did she say?" I asked John inquisitively.

"She has gone to see if she can find out anything for us," he told me.

Within a few moments, the receptionist returned and informed us that I would be seen shortly.

"Would you like a drink of water, or is there anything else that I can get you?" she asked.

"No thank you," I replied.

The one thing I wanted she could not give me; my discharge from hospital.

I was surprised to find Professor Cooke who was in charge of the breast cancer clinic approach us. Instantly he apologised for the time it was taking for me to be seen. He then went on to explain that I would not only be seeing one of the doctors on his team, but I would also be seeing an oncologist. Slightly puzzled, I looked at John. I hadn't been told by Jean or the ward sister that I would be seeing an oncologist. I had assumed I was only going to the clinic to be checked over before being discharged.

I was now beginning to become nervous at the thought of seeing this specialist. I had never given a thought to the possibility that things would start moving that quickly. To be honest, I was rather dumfounded and had only just got my head around the fact that I might have needed this form of treatment; now, here I was, waiting to be told all about the ins and outs of it.

Not long after, I was quickly examined by a member of Professor Cooke's team. How I wished that it had been Alison my surgeon. Alas, it was not to be. After telling me that I was now officially discharged, the young male doctor that had examined me then handed me a slip of paper.

"That is when we next want to see you at the clinic. If you take it to the receptionist, she will note it on an appointment card for you," he said.

"One down, one to go," I thought to myself.

Just as I was about to take a seat in the waiting area, my name was once again being called. On entering the consultation room, both John and I were met by a man of around sixty who introduced himself as Dr Scott. He told us that he was the head of the oncologist team that would be dealing with my treatment. Within minutes of entering this room, he then explained that it was felt that I would benefit from a 6-month course of treatment, all of course news to me. What came next even startled me more.

"After reviewing your case, however, I feel it would be advisable that you also have a 3-month course of a chemotherapy drug known as Doxorubicin. This would be given prior to the 6-month course originally planned."

That was 9 months of chemotherapy treatment in total. I could not believe my ears. I did not think it was possible to give someone this form of treatment for that length of time. How the hell was I going to survive 9 whole months of ongoing chemotherapy? I got to my feet and began to rock back and forth from one foot to the other, hoping it would help ease the pain that was now affecting my ability to focus on what was being said.

"Mrs Gallagher, breast cancer is a form of cancer that we know can emit small cancerous seeds to other areas in the body. Given that we are unable to determine if this has happened or not, I feel it would be better not to take any chances. It's like, for example, increasing an insurance policy to cover every possible eventuality," this doctor explained.

I remember thinking to myself that those were the very same words I had read on one of the fact sheets on chemotherapy treatments that Jean had given me only a few days earlier.

Dr Scott continued by explaining that Doxorubicin chemotherapy was not a particularly pleasant form of treatment.

"I know it will be hard going," he said.

What could I say? I was no expert in the field of chemotherapy, so how could I make the decision on whether or not I should have this treatment? My mind raced as all the information I was being given swirled around in my head.

"So if you were in my position, would you have this treatment?" I asked the doctor.

Telling me he would was enough for me. This man knew what he was talking about and obviously had my best interests at heart, so I accepted his advice and agreed to go through the 3-mouth course of Doxorubicin chemotherapy.

You hear so many stories/myths of people having to endure horrendous chemotherapy treatments when all the while the doctors know that the patient is dying. How often have you heard the words, "They were only using him as a guinea pig; they shouldn't have put him through that"? I must admit these very thoughts crossed my mind. I couldn't help myself.

"You are a very brave woman, Mrs. Gallagher," the doctor told me.

"No, not me," I replied.

As I left the clinic, I was handed yet another piece of paper, this time for my next oncology appointment date.

Handing it to the receptionist, I was promptly given yet another appointment card.

In the car on our way home, I mulled over what had been said at my consultation when John broke my chain of thought.

"What are you thinking about?" he asked me.

"I'm trying hard to take in what is in front of me. The thought of the next 9 months scares the hell out of me," I told him. "Then after that I have to go through, I think, 30 treatments of radiotherapy. That will be nearly a whole year," I lamented.

"Don't worry. I know you; if anyone can get through this, you can Roseann."

I wasn't that convinced.

Chapter Nine

Home at Last

That night was not a good one for me. I was in a lot of pain and just could not find a comfortable position to sit in on any of the two sofas in our living room. John tried everything, from putting lots of cushions and pillows around me, to getting a heated pad and placing it where I felt the pain was most severe, but nothing seemed to work. In the end, I took a sleeping tablet with my painkillers and went to bed in the hope of sleeping.

Waking up after a few hours, I found that John was lying beside me fast asleep. Not wanting to wake him, I slowly and gradually got myself out of the bed. I felt so sore. Trying to get from a lying position to an upright one was terrible. Inside, my body felt like two pieces of Velcro detaching. I finally got to my feet, made my way downstairs and put on the kettle to make myself a cup of tea.

Sitting with my tea in our lounge, I felt so alone. It's amazing how situations seem so much worse in the middle of the night. I began to go over in my mind all the treatments that I would have to endure.

Like everyone else, I was well aware of all the horror stories regarding chemotherapy treatment; statements such as "Oh, it was terrible; he went through torture", or "She was constantly being sick; never had her head out of the toilet bowl" and "What was it all for? He died anyway". I think you get the picture.

Then there was the radiotherapy treatment. Was it going

to hurt? Would I be left with horrific burns? Just thinking about those treatments brought me out in a sweat.

I drank my tea quickly, wanting to get back to bed, if only to rid me of the terrible feeling of being alone. I also prayed that sleep would come not long after to help me escape temporarily from these horrible thoughts that just would not stop crowding my mind. John was still fast asleep as I slowly lowered myself back into bed and, thank God, fell asleep not long after.

The following morning I awoke to find that John was already up and about. Surprisingly I hadn't even felt him get out of the bed. I felt sore and rather stiff and any thoughts I had of getting up were hampered by the dreaded thought of having to get myself into the sitting position. I hated that awful feeling of detachment inside my chest; it was almost as if things were knitting together only to be torn apart again when I moved in a certain way. I shouted to John to come up and help me. I hoped that by physically helping me to sit up, he would hopefully help to alleviate the direct strain on my body. What a difference it made; through this small action, the pain and discomfort that I had been experiencing was reduced dramatically.

It felt as if I had taken one step forward when discharged from hospital and two steps back since my return home. It took me ages to get dressed and just as long to get myself downstairs. I gave a sigh of relief on entering our lounge and finding a hot cup of tea that John had made sitting on the table next to one of our sofas. It was great to be home.

My mum and dad popped in to see how I was doing later that day and stayed for a few hours. That was like the icing on the cake for me, as I hadn't seen my dad since my admission to hospital. He's terrified of them you see.

"I will see you when you get home daughter; your mother will keep me informed," he told me the day prior to my admission.

It was and had always been something that often made my family and I laugh; the fact that my dad was scared stiff when it came to hospitals. We could never get him into one.

The rest of that day was really quite uneventful. I spent most of my time taking things easy and having lots of little naps. It's amazing how quickly tiredness overwhelms you after a period in hospital.

The following day, I awoke feeling as if I could have taken on the world. The previous night had been the first time in ages that I had actually had a full night's sleep. I was so pleased that I even managed to potter slowly around the house. As the day went by, I just kept feeling better and better and after a nap in the afternoon, I asked John if he would take me out for a breath of fresh air, to which he agreed, after forceful persuasion.

"We can surprise your mum," I told him, as we both got into the car.

John's mum lived on the other side of town.

"Just a nice run in the car and a short visit, that's all," I told him.

His expression told me that he thought it a bad idea. I think he felt I was doing too much too soon. I reassured him that I would be alright.

We had brought pillows from the house to position in front of my body to act like a cushion, as well as to prevent the seatbelt from touching my body. It was a bit hair-raising and I must admit I could feel myself tense up in apprehension as John clicked my seatbelt into position. I need not have worried though, for all in all I was rather comfy. I did enjoy that run in the car. I felt human again; just an ordinary everyday person going about her business.

John's mum was over the moon at seeing us turn up on her doorstep. As we chatted away, she went on about how she could come and look after me if I needed her. Truth be told, I didn't think I would feel comfortable at having her wash my underwear and things, if you know what I mean. She most probably would have felt the same if the boot had been on the other foot. I didn't reply to her suggestion, hoping her words would fade into the background without further comment. After about an hour tiredness overcame me once more and we quickly said our goodbyes.

By the time we arrived home, I think I was just about ready for dropping. All I wanted to do was get out of my clothes and into my nightgown. I knew that would make me feel a whole lot better. As it was still early evening, I decided to try and rest on one of our sofas rather than my bed. I hated being stuck upstairs at times.

Snuggled up comfortably, I suggested to John that he should go down to our local and chill with a nice cold beer. He had been going at it non-stop whilst I was in hospital and also since I had got home. He needed a break, a chance just to relax. I told him that I would most likely sleep whilst he was away and that if he put everything that I needed on a small table next to me, I would be fine. So there I was lying quite comfortably on the sofa, telephone at hand in case I needed John and everything else that we thought I might need on the table next to me. With that, I kissed John goodbye and told him to enjoy his time out.

I must have nodded off not long after John had left, but had been woken by the sound of the telephone ring. Lifting the cordless handset, the voice on the other end was that of a very good friend.

"I just thought I would give you a quick call to see how you are doing," she said.

"Getting there slowly, but surely," I told her.

Changing the subject, she then went on to tell me that she had got herself a new boyfriend.

"Oh Roseann, he's really nice," she excitedly told me.

I was now wishing I hadn't answered the telephone. The last thing I needed was to listen to my friend go on about some guy she had met. There was no stopping her as she went into great detail about how they had met and how much they had in common. I tried to make short, positive comments, but all the while wishing she would get off the telephone. Any other time, I would have been only too happy to listen to her talk about this guy, but not now, not so soon after being discharged from hospital.

Out of the blue she asked me if she could bring him up to my house to meet me. I couldn't believe what she was asking. Being a nurse and a woman, I thought that she would have instinctively known that the last thing I wanted to do was meet a stranger, not only that but a stranger of the opposite sex. Knowing my friend as I did, I knew that she would have already told him all about my breast cancer. How could she not see that I would feel uncomfortable sitting in the company of this guy, knowing that he would be fully aware that I had just had my breast removed? I wondered how she could be so insensitive and I could feel myself becoming increasingly annoyed as our conversation continued.

To add insult to injury, my friend then went on to tell me about how her new boyfriend's mum had cancer and how gravely ill she was. It was as if she seemed to think that by

Cancer No Not Me!

telling me this, it made it then alright for him to come to my house. I curtly told her that I was not up to visitors, especially ones that I did not know and that I would telephone her soon. I was numbed by the whole experience.

The last thing I needed was a full blown conversation about another person's cancer. It was taking me all my time to try and cope with my own situation. I couldn't afford to lose focus. I knew that by being the type of person that I was, I would have taken all this woman's problems onto my shoulders as if they were mine and for my own sanity I needed all my own strength and energy for myself if I were to successfully fight my own cancer.

What my friend had just done unnerved me and all the feelings of vulnerability that I had tried to put from my mind came flooding back. Did cancer always mean impending death? I was beginning to doubt my ability to beat this awful disease.

The conversation with my friend had upset me that much that in the end I telephoned our local pub. I had to speak to John. On telling him all about my conversation with my friend, he was furious.

"I'll be straight home," he told me, but I didn't want that. I only wanted to hear him tell me that everything would be alright, which he did. After speaking to him, I felt so much better. Putting my friend's telephone call to the back of my mind, I return to watching television.

About an hour after my upset over my friend's call, the door bell rang. Was I ever going to get any peace that night? Struggling to get onto my side, I then had to try and roll onto my knees in order to stand up. It certainly wasn't easy and without John to help me, the Velcro detaching feeling in my chest was excruciating as I tried to sit up. Eventually though, I got myself onto my feet and made my way slowly to the front door.

I could not believe it; as I opened the door slightly ajar, there stood my friend with a bouquet in hand. Next to her was a guy whom I assumed was her new boyfriend.

"Surprise!" she said.

I could have killed her as I stood in the doorway trying desperately to hide the shape of my body. I felt so uncomfortable standing there, knowing that under my nightdress was one large boob on the right of my body and one great big bloody hollow space on the left. Taking the few steps up into the hallway, my friend left me no other option but to let them both come in. I tried desperately to dash for my housecoat whilst holding my nightdress away from my body in an attempt to mask my surgery, all the while feeling that this guy could see every contour of my body. It felt as if I was never going to get my housecoat on, as I struggled with the arm holes. After finally managing to do so, I then sat down on the sofa, pulling the quilt that John had brought down from the bedroom up over my body, almost as if it were my shield.

Picking up the telephone once again, I dialled the number of the pub to speak to John, this time to ask him to come home. There was no way I could face sitting with them on my own.

The remainder of their visit was awful as my friend openly asked me very personal questions in front of this stranger, apparently oblivious to the effect that it was having on me. I was so glad when John walked through the door and came to my rescue.

Do you know that after that night I could not bring myself to speak with my friend; she had really hurt me by not understanding how her actions made me feel. It got to the stage where I refused to take all her telephone calls and I couldn't even think about her without feeling rage at what she had done. It took me a year before I did eventually speak to her. Then I told her how badly her actions had affected me. She told me she hadn't the slightest inclination that I felt that way, telling me of how she was so truly sorry for the upset she had caused. Our relationship suffered badly over that incident and it took a long time before I could put it all behind me.

Two weeks had passed since my discharge from hospital and it was a day away from my next arranged appointment to see Alison at the breast clinic. Over that time I had slowly became stronger within myself, although despite the wider range of movement, my arm remained very weak and had no power in it at all. My left armpit and the surrounding area felt numb and the rest of the area around my surgery site felt electrified. The detaching Velcro feeling had thankfully subsided, although on occasions I would experience short, sharp shooting pains. I remained edgy when anyone came close to me, terrified that they would bump into me and for that reason I was also reluctant to go outside, that is unless travelling by car.

Lying down also caused me problems. It would take what seemed like forever to get myself lowered and then it would take even longer for me to eventually find a position that I found comfortable. Getting back up again was still a performance and it would sometimes take at least 2–3 attempts before I successfully managed to get myself in an upright sitting position. Most of the time I would become frustrated at not being able to do much of anything and

Cancer No Not Me!

other times I would experience emotions and feelings that I could not control, like panic attacks at the thought that I was near death. I would also, without any warning, find myself in uncontrollable floods of tears and no matter how much reassurance I would receive from John or Billy, I would find it impossible to stop.

Alison was at her desk as both John and I entered the consultation room in the breast clinic. Jean was also present.

"I see that you have met Dr Scott, your oncologist and he has discussed with you the fact that he feels it is in your best interests that you also have 3 months' treatment of Doxorubicin Chemotherapy," she said, as she looked through my hospital case notes.

She then asked how I had been keeping and after being told of the difficulties I had been experiencing, she told me how she was well aware that my recovery would be hard.

"I had to take away so much of the muscle, tissue and skin that had surrounded your breast," she informed me.

At least I now understood why I had been experiencing so many problems.

Although frightened at what I might hear, I had to ask Alison if she would truthfully tell me my chances of survival. Nervously I began to speak.

"Alison, what are my chances of survival? The reason I ask is that I am the type of person that needs to know exactly where they stand in order to muster the energy to fight."

There, I had said it. I sat anxiously waiting for my surgeon to reply.

"Are you absolutely sure that you want me to answer that question?" she asked me.

"Yes," I confirmed.

Firstly, Alison made it quite clear that it was only facts and figures that she could quote and that even they were not a solid ground to go on.

"Even with all the technology that we have, cancer still, to this day, can surprise us by reacting in a totally different way than even we anticipated. You can never be sure what will happen sometimes. Everyone reacts totally differently. It's an individual thing and one person whom we thought would have benefited greatly from the treatment they are given, dumfounds us by reacting in at totally different way from that which we anticipated. In the same instance, you may come up against a case were the person in question may have a very poor prognosis, but baffles even us in a professional sense by reacting favourably to a treatment that we may have thought would not have given a great result."

Her words did not change my mind. I still needed her to explain to me how she felt personally with regard to my future.

"I understand you can obviously only give me statistics, but please I need you to be honest with me," I told her.

Alison went on to tell me that were I not to have the planned treatments of chemotherapy, radiotherapy and the ongoing drug therapy in the form of Tamoxifen, the statistics would be around a 20% chance of surviving 5 years. That was a blow. She then continued by telling me that with chemotherapy and radiotherapy treatments, the statistics would then increase to about a 40% chance of surviving 5 years.

"If you then take into the equation the drug Tamoxifen, that would add a further 8% to your life expectancy," she concluded.

So all in all, what I was being told was that I had a 48%

chance of living for 5 years. That was hard to digest. I honestly did not expect to be told that, statistically, my life expectancy was so poor.

I tried not to show just how deeply the news had affected me by saying something like, "Now I know what I'm up against. I can at least visualise what I am fighting."

After a momentary silence, Alison totally changed the subject and to tell you the truth I was relieved. If our conversation on my mortality had continued, I think I would have truly fallen to pieces in front of them all. John squeezed my hand tightly to let me know that he was there for me.

"I want to talk to you about something known as a Hickman line," Alison continued, explaining that this was a procedure where a line is fed directly into the bloodstream via a vein that is situated near the lung. "Oh no, not more surgery," I thought as I listened. "I feel this is something that you would benefit from due to the fact that you have very poor veins," she said.

Now I knew that was very true given that every time I was required to give a sample of blood, my veins more often than not would collapse and instead of a flow of blood from the arm to the syringe, mine would slowly drip and I would then have to go through the whole procedure all over again; sometimes up to as many as eight times before a sample of blood could be successfully obtained.

Alison also informed me that my impending chemotherapy treatment could be given via a Hickman line.

"Many people find that the further into their treatment they get, the harder it becomes to get a healthy vein. In your case, your veins are poor to start with, plus the fact that your chemotherapy treatment is over quite a lengthy period of time, so I believe you would benefit by having this procedure. It would also eliminate the problems of endless unsuccessful attempts to have blood taken from your body," she finished.

How could I say no? This was obviously something that I needed to have done in order to ensure that my bloods could be monitored and also so that I could be given the much needed chemotherapy treatment.

"What does it entail?" I asked her.

She told me that it was not a lengthy procedure, but she did highlight that it was one that had to be done in an operating theatre.

"You will only have to attend the day ward and will be able to go home within a few hours," she said reassuringly.

It was then simply a case of setting a date. After looking at her dairy, Alison suggested a week that Friday, only 9 days away.

Again, so much had happened at my clinic appointment. Not only did I have the worry of my life expectancy on my mind, but I also had to try and cope with the thought of having to go back to theatre. Where was it all going to end? Would I have to go through all this for nothing and die anyway? That was a question I knew no one could answer for me. Leaving the clinic that day, I had a very strange experience, determination from I don't know where; an overwhelming feeling of wanting to fight and believe that I could beat the cancer. "I will fight this all the way," I told myself. "I am not going to die. I am too bloody young and have so much to live for."

Over the run-up to my next hospital admission, I tried hard to eat well and rest. I was determined to give myself all the important things I thought my body would need to successfully recover from the major surgery that I had gone through, not once, but twice over a very short period of time. My body must have been thinking to itself "What the hell is going on here?"

The feelings of drive and determination I harboured made me believe I could move mountains. I had made up my mind that I would face one day at a time. I was no longer going to wallow in self pity, promising myself that there would be no hiding away for me. I would make damn sure that the people I knew would see me regularly. If I distanced myself, I would be unable to cope with the stares, reactions or shocked looks from people at seeing the dramatic changes in my appearance as my treatment progressed and my hair fell out. I needed to stay focused and could not take the chance of letting anything, or anyone, knock my confidence. I had decided that I would make sure that I continued to visit our local pub on a regular basis as a way of keeping in contact with those who knew me. I knew it would be hard and a struggle at times, but I was determined to do it, even if it meant John having to drive me the 20 yards it took to get there.

Another thing that would help me move up my imaginary ladder of success, step by step, was to set myself small achievable goals, an idea I had taken from a friend who had fought and won a battle with cancer.

"They help keep you strong and make you more determined in your fight to survive," he had told me.

Chapter Ten

Out, In, Out

John had arranged to go on a weekend away with the Territorial Army. We had both been medics in the Royal Army Medical Corps and although I had given it up, John was still very much involved. The weekend was obligatory and had been planned long before any mention had been made of me having to go back into hospital to have a Hickman line put in place. I had told John that I hadn't wanted him to cancel his weekend away, explaining I would be alright, as I had Billy and the rest of my family to look after me. So, with it all arranged, we only hoped that everything would go as planned.

I was due to go into the day ward early morning, so taking everything into consideration – the going to theatre, having the line put in place and then the few hours that they would want to monitor me afterwards – we had worked out that John would still have plenty of time to get ready and then drive himself to the barracks where the weekend was due to take place.

In the car on my way to hospital that Friday morning, I felt nervous and certainly did not want to face yet another trip to the operating theatre, but what could I do? I reminded myself that I was determined to fight all the way.

As parking was difficult and there was no real reason for John to come to the day ward with me, as I believed I would be going to theatre shortly after I had arrived, I told him that he should just drop me off at the ward.

Cancer No Not Me!

"That way," I explained, "you can then get started on the clothes you need to iron for your weekend away. Don't worry I will be fine," I reassured him.

Walking into the ward, I was surprised at how fresh and modern it was considering it was housed in a very old building. After giving the nurse at the main desk of the ward my details, I was then shown to a lounge area to wait for further instructions.

Sitting there in that lounge my eyes began to wander. I began taking in all the furnishings and surroundings. I could not help but notice that a lot of the furnishings in the lounge had been donated by family members in memory of their loved ones. That made me feel very unsettled and I instinctively began to feel myself becoming frightened and upset over this. Don't get me wrong. I knew in reality this was an amazing thing; families of loved ones who had died from cancer donating a piece of furnishing or pictures in their memory. But given that I had been diagnosed with cancer and was still very much alive, these things made me feel uneasy. I became more and more frightened the more I noticed yet another donation.

I had always found it hard to take in, or even comprehend, that I could possibly be so ill, but looking over all those personalised plaques that were individually attached to each donated item, hit me hard. It felt as if someone had come right up to me and slapped me hard across the face, almost as if to tell me, "Now do you believe how ill you are?" It was truly unnerving. I promised myself there and then that I would make sure my family understood that I did not want to be remembered in this way should I die.

Some time had passed and I was still sitting in the same seat within the ward lounge waiting to be told what I should do. I felt as if they had forgotten about me. I hadn't taken the usual bag you would prepare when going into hospital, as I knew that I would have to wear the standard hospital theatre gown and as it was only a day ward, I would not be staying in overnight.

A few hours later and I still hadn't seen a soul, apart from the nurse at the desk when I had come in that morning and an older man who had come into the lounge to wait whilst his wife was being discharged.

I watched the usual daytime TV rubbish and looked at countless out of date magazines that were spread out across a table. Lunchtime arrived and I was still no further forward. I had phoned John on a few occasions since my arrival at the ward, most of the time just to say the same thing: "I'm still waiting."

Eventually, a nurse did come to see me to inform me that it would now be late afternoon before I would be going down to theatre. On asking her why it was taking so long, explaining I had been under the impression that I would have been on my way back home, she replied that there must have been crossed wires over timings because according to her I was the last person on her list for theatre that day.

Again I telephoned John. By this time I was on the verge of crying.

"Why can't anything ever be simple in my life?" I griped.

Continuing, I told him to carry on as planned, telling him that if I wasn't ready to go home before he had to leave for his weekend away, then Billy could pick me up when I was ready to go home.

"No, I'll cancel the weekend," he told me.

"Look, I will be alright; stop worrying," I reassured him.

Then, promising to keep in touch, I told John I loved him and said my goodbyes.

It was around 4pm before I was taken to have my Hickman line put in place. As I arrived in theatre, I was met by Alison.

"This procedure is done under local anaesthetic," she told me.

"Great," I thought to myself, as my nerves heightened.

Alison continued by explaining briefly what she was going to do.

"There will be a lot of manoeuvring and pulling and tugging, but you shouldn't feel any pain," she told me.

"Thank God for that," I remember thinking to myself.

It was also explained to me that at some point during this procedure the operating table would have to be manoeuvred in such a way that my head would be positioned near to the floor and my feet would be up in the air. In other words, I would be upside down, something that I found quite amusing and a thought that momentarily managed to sidetrack me from my anxiety. To tell you the truth, I didn't really know if Alison was actually serious or if she was joking. I laughed nervously anyway.

Taking a deep breath, I closed my eyes and tried hard to focus on the sound of the monitors that were attached to my body, which by now were making a continual bleeping noise. Other noises began to creep in, such as the everyday conversation of the medical staff. They spoke of what they were going to be doing on their weekend off and how one of them had bought a new pair of shoes. It's strange, but I felt almost embarrassed at listening in on a conversation that did not concern me.

During the procedure, the operating table on which I lay did indeed continually move and at one point it felt as if I was on a ride at the fairground. True to Alison's word, I did find myself positioned with my feet in the air and head to the floor whilst having my arm pulling rather firmly to hold it in a certain position by one of the assisting nurses.

Having this procedure done was rather nerve racking, not knowing what to expect next. However, I must stress that it wasn't too bad and apart from the small sting of the injection given to me at the start of the procedure, it was a totally painless experience.

Arriving back on the ward, a nurse instructed the porter who had brought me from theatre to take me to a bed in the farthest bay of the ward, whilst she followed on. Given that it was now almost 6pm, I knew it would be pointless phoning home to speak to John, since he would already be on his way to his weekend with the Territorial Army.

Once on my ward bed, I took a deep breath, glad that the day was now behind me and that it would only be a matter of hours before I would be once again in the safety of my own home. Funny how you always feel better in your own environment isn't it? I did think of telephoning my son, but thought it best to wait until I had a rough idea of when I would be discharged. I took a quick peek under my hospital gown and checked the site where the tube had been inserted into my body more closely. I noted that it was only a small incision at the top of my right breast and not far from my collar bone. Two stitches were visible, obviously to secure the Hickman line tube in position. I also noticed that there was a small continuous trickle of blood coming from the wound, but dismissed this as nothing, assuming that this was normal and it would settle.

I lay back and tried to rest, but as the anaesthetic began to wear off, I began to feel sore around and inside the wound. That didn't concern me too much because I would have expected some discomfort, given the pulling and prodding that had been done to my body whilst in theatre.

There were two other female patients in the bay with me and on speaking with the patient in the bed that directly faced mine, I found out that she had Hodgkin's Disease. She did appear rather poorly, but I would never have dreamed of telling her that. In the short time that I had been in the ward since my return from theatre, she must have been visited at least four times by the doctor that was looking after her.

The other female patient was asleep, totally unaware that there was a conversation going on.

"She is very ill. Her cancer has spread and there is nothing that can be done for her other than to make her as comfortable as possible," the Hodgkin's patient informed me.

I looked at the other woman as she lay so very still. My heart went out to her. No wonder she was out cold. I surmised that it was probably a high dose of pain medication that was making her sleep so soundly.

"Well at least while she is asleep she will be pain free," I found myself voicing to the other woman.

As time went by, I was examined twice in the space of about twenty minutes by one of the nurses.

"When will I be discharged? I asked her on both occasions.

I was so desperate to go home, but the nurse made no mention of when that time would be, opting only to focus all her attention on the fact that my wound continued to bleed, even if it was only slightly.

"I will come back and check on you again shortly," she told me before disappearing.

The fact that time continued to pass and still I was no further forward began to irritate me. I looked at my watch and noted that it was now 7pm. Any longer and it would be visiting time. Now that was something that made me feel uncomfortable, given that I had not brought any personal items with me and was still in a hospital gown. Wondering if I could now get dressed, I waited for the nurse to return to ask her. The last thing I wanted was to sit in a hospital ward full of visitors looking like a pauper.

"Can I get dressed now? I asked the nurse upon her return.

To my surprise she told me she would rather I stayed in a hospital gown, going on to explain that she felt it would be much easier to monitor my wound. Oh how I now wished I had brought a toilet bag and nightdress with me, a "just in case" measure, as this was now turning into exactly one of those occasions.

Asking the nurse if I could get out of bed as I needed to telephone my son, I began to swing my legs out of the bed. The relief I felt at being told that I could get out of that bed was phenomenal; it was as if I had been set free. I couldn't wait to get to the telephone, desperate to hear a familiar voice. Hearing Billy's voice only made the stress that I had felt over the whole day come to a head. I could now feel myself close to tears.

"I don't know when I will be discharged. Nobody in here seems to know and I feel like a pauper stuck in this hospital gown. I did ask if I could get dressed, but they advised me not to, something to do with wanting to monitor the slight bleeding from my wound," I told my son.

As our telephone conversation continued, I could feel my emotions heighten and before long that awful feeling of vulnerability overpowered me; the feeling of having absolutely no control over my own life. I was in the hands of strangers and that scared me. Again, it was fear of the unknown or of what would happen next

"Look mum, calm down. After I have finished speaking to you, I will telephone the ward and find out what's happening," he reassured me. "I will then put some toiletries and a couple of your own nightdresses in a bag and bring it up to you," he continued.

Making my way back to my bed in the ward, I felt a bit breathless. Slowing my pace, I told myself that it was most probably exhaustion that was making me feel this way. Once back in bed, I fanned myself with a magazine.

"You can hardly get a breath in here," I commented to the woman I had been speaking to earlier.

Once again the nurse returned to check on me. However, before checking my wound as she had on all the other occasions, she said, "You appear to be a bit breathless Mrs Gallagher." Before I could reply, she continued, "I think it's best that I get one of the doctors to check you over. Best to be on the safe side."

"Yet another hold up," I thought to myself.

"It's only because it's so warm in here," I told her, in the hope that she would accept this as the cause of my breathlessness. My attempts at trying to make her see that there was a simple reason for the change in my breathing fell on deaf ears as once again she repeated that she thought it best that a doctor check me out.

Shortly after, a young man approached me and introduced himself as the doctor on call for the ward.

"Do you mind if I have a look at your Hickman line and listen to your chest?" he asked me.

After examining me fully, the doctor then went on to inform me that he suspected that I could possibly have a collapsed lung. I was totally shocked. I just could not believe what was happening.

"I would like to send you for a chest x-ray to confirm or eliminate my diagnosis," he informed me.

Cancer No Not Me!

Sitting on top of the bed, I tried to absorb the news. First I went through surgery for breast cancer only to find that I had to go through yet further major surgery only weeks later. I was told that I might need radiotherapy, only to find that in the space of a few days the goal posts changed and I also required two different chemotherapy treatments and an ongoing drug. Now, I had only come into hospital for a simple procedure, only to discover that I had a suspected collapsed lung and a wound that would not stop bleeding. To top it all, as the visitors arrived, I instantly recognised a young man who had come in to visit the lady that was so gravely ill. He was one of my husband's old work colleagues. It was awful sitting there trying to be inconspicuous. The last thing I wanted was for him to realise who I was, not only because I did not want him to know I was being treated for cancer, but also because I knew the person he was visiting was seriously ill. It was even harder when I heard him call her "Mother".

By the time Billy had arrived at the ward, I had been down for an x-ray and back. Now all I had to do was wait for the doctor to come back and tell me the results.

"I telephoned Gran and told her you were still in hospital. She is on her way up," Billy said.

I would have probably not have told her, as I wouldn't have wanted to worry her, but now that she knew, I was glad she was on her way.

The doctor appeared and took a seat by my bed. He then explained to us that my chest x-rays showed that my lung had collapsed.

"I would be much happier if you were to stay in hospital overnight," he told me, as tears ran down my face. "Mrs Gallagher, I must stress to you how important it is that your condition be monitored closely. In my opinion you risk jeopardising your health further should you go home tonight," he said.

"Mum, it's only one night. I've got everything you need with me," my son prompted, obviously keen that I take the doctor's advice.

So that was it, I would spend the night in hospital.

When my mother arrived with my sister Iris, her first reaction on seeing me was to give me a right telling off at not contacting her. Her second was then to proceed to empty the contents of a bag she had brought with her; fruit, biscuits, sandwiches and toiletries. I think she must have brought everything but the kitchen sink with her that night, not that I was complaining. I even started to feel a bit more like my old myself now that I had some of my family around me. Looking from one to the other, I thought to myself how truly blessed I was.

Ironically, would you believe it, my hospital stay lasted for the entire weekend. However, all in all, it wasn't too bad. I learned not to look at the loving memory plaques on the walls and tried instead to focus only on getting well.

What also made my stay in that ward so much easier was the kindness and understanding shown to me by one of the night nurses. She was a lovely person who took the time to personally share a few precious moments with all of her patients individually. For me she was like a tower of strength, taking the time to show her genuine concern at my diagnosis and the mammoth road of treatment I had in front of me. It's truly amazing how one individual can make such a difference to one's life; she certainly was and is one of God's Earth angels and a credit to her profession.

Chapter Eleven

The Run Up

I had received an appointment to meet with the chemotherapy nurse who would be looking after me for the duration of my treatment. I was to attend a clinic that was situated below the ward that I had been in previously when having my Hickman line put in place. It felt strange to experience no apprehension about the meeting, considering the way things had been going for me. Maybe it was because I was not actually going for any form of treatment, just a general introduction and a talk about what it actually entailed.

The clinic was bright and fresh, but thankfully without the "In Loving Memory" furnishings. My mother accompanied me that day and was also surprised not to be greeted by gloomy surroundings. The receptionist appeared to be very nice and instantly smiled at us as I handed her my appointment letter. Chirpily she told me to take a seat before telephoning through to the nurse to let her know that I had arrived. There were a few people sitting in the waiting area. One person my eyes instantly registered was a young woman of about 30 who appeared rather poorly; very gaunt and with no hair. I remember instantly feeling sorry for her as she looked as if she had been to hell and back.

I consciously tried hard not to let my thoughts of my impending treatment overwhelm me, trying only to remain focused on why I had come to the clinic that day. A short while later, a young woman walked from – what I assumed was – another part of the clinic and called my name. My poor mum was up off her seat like a shot and at the ready. She tried to appear in control, but I knew she was more nervous than I at being there that day. The woman instantly introduced herself as Veronica, explaining that she was the nurse who would be looking after me. She asked that we follow her and began to walk in the direction from which she had come.

It was definitely an eye opener to find that within such a short distance from the main reception, we were slap bang in the middle of a very large, open spaced area, filled with large reclining chairs against every possible wall space, with the exception of an area taken up by two hospital beds, one of which had the screens fully drawn. I found myself amazed by the number of people that were there, as my eyes tried to take in all the things that appeared to be going on. There were at least eight or nine men and women, all sitting on reclining chairs, who appeared to be in the process of having chemotherapy treatment via drugs that hung from drip stands and ran from tubes directly into their bloodstream. The reason I surmised this was because some of the bags containing fluid were covered by bright red bags with hazardous signs emblazoned all over them.

There were around three other nurses in attendance. Two appeared to be busily monitoring everything and another was in the process of skilfully extracting blood from one of the female patients. Everything was so public.

On offering us both two unoccupied seats in a corner of the room, Veronica apologetically informed us that the room that she had hoped we could have for a private chat was engaged, apparently by a doctor and one of the patients.

"Would you mind if we spoke here?" she asked.

To be honest, her request didn't really bother me, as it wasn't as if I was going to be physically examined, plus I assumed that there was not that much we had to discuss. The extreme lack of privacy that the patients had to endure did shock me, although I must stress that none of the patients appeared fazed by this. Whether it was because they felt more secure in numbers, or because they had no choice other than to accept the situation I don't know, but apart from the small room mentioned by Veronica that was presently occupied, there appeared to be nowhere for patients to be seen or examined privately. The only visual privacy afforded were the screens that could be pulled around the two beds, but even then they weren't that practical, because everyone on the outside side of the screens could still hear the full conversation that went on behind them.

My mother's eyes moved in the direction of the bed that was screened off and I knew by her reaction that she too thought that it wasn't fair to the patient behind the screen, who at that point was having a very personal discussion about their treatment and health issues.

Veronica distracted me from my analysis of the clinic as she began to go through my personal details; what surgery I had undergone, my name and address, next of kin and all the usual questions one is asked when in hospital. Talking about the benefits of having a Hickman line, she highlighted the difficulties of finding veins in chemotherapy patients. "More often than not we have to get the patient to sit with their hand in a bucket of hot water to help raise their veins," she said.

Thoroughly, Veronica described the two different kinds of chemotherapy treatments that I would be having and told me how patients also received different drugs to take home with them after receiving their treatment; anti-sickness drugs and medication to help prevent mouth ulcers, apparently a common ailment in chemotherapy patients. They might also be given other drugs if required, such as remedies for constipation.

"Will I lose my hair?" I anxiously asked her, although I don't know why because it had already been explained to me that I would by my oncologist. Maybe I was clutching at very fine straws and hoped that this would not be the case. Veronica told me that the chemotherapy treatment Doxorubicin definitely caused hair loss. My heart sank at the realisation that this treatment would be my first course of chemotherapy and that the experience of baldness would be soon very much part of my life. Quickly I erased these thoughts from my mind, telling myself that I would cross that bridge when I came to it.

My meeting with Veronica didn't last much longer after that. As there were no other pressing questions that I felt I needed answered at that point, I said my goodbyes and walked arm in arm with my mother as we made our way out of the clinic. Veronica's parting words of "See you soon Roseann" rang in my ears. Strangely, the hairs on my back stood tall.

Things seemed to now be going well for me. My Hickman line appeared to be working as it should and most of the time I found that I was unaware that I had two tubes permanently protruding from my body.

I had now been assigned a district nurse who visited my home every few days to do what is known as a line flush. Basically, this was a procedure were the nurse would inject a syringe of saline into each of my lines in order to maintain a clear line and reduce the possibility of blockages; all very painless and nothing to write home about. My house was quickly becoming like a medical supply store, stockpiled with dressings, syringes and the like, something John and I often joked about.

I had also been prescribed a daily dose of Warfarin, a blood thinning drug to reduce the possibility of blood clots and to aid in the maintenance of a blockage free Hickman line. There were no side effects associated with this form of medication; however, there was a need to monitor the dosage and I would regularly require blood tests to ensure that it had not become too thin. This test was totally pain free and done in a matter of minutes by extracting a blood sample from my Hickman line. I could now understand my surgeon's explanation of the benefits of having a Hickman line, not only because it eliminated the need for me to have needles constantly plunged into my body, but also because it strangely enough contributed in expanding my social connections by providing me with the company of a district nurse on a regular basis; a Godsend on the days I felt down or weepy.

My district nurse's name was Isabell Munro and the minute I met her I knew we would click. I so looked forward to her visits and viewed them as a social event rather than a medical necessity. She was – and is – an amazing person who became a big part of my life and played many roles; a nurse in the first instance, but also a confidante and advisor. I don't know what I would have done at times if I had not had Isabell to talk to about my deepest fears and concerns. We spent many hours talking in great depth as she went through the process of flushing my Hickman line. Even when she had completed the task she was there to do, she would make a point of taking the time to listen and advise me on something that may have been troubling me on that particular day. Nothing was ever too much trouble for her and on occasions she would even collect my prescription to save John from having to go to the surgery. I'm sure most days she worked through her lunch breaks, if not to assist me in some way, then to assist one of her other many patients.

Looking at my body in the full length mirror in my bedroom one day, I could not help but feel utter disgust at the horrible reflection that looked back at me. I felt like a freak with a horrible deformity and wondered whether I would ever feel feminine again; I certainly didn't that day, the day I had taken the first real look at myself since having my surgery. As I stood there naked from top to toe, I slowly and gradually scanned my body. I didn't feel like a woman anymore, which lead on to thoughts of my future sex life. I certainly didn't feel in the least bit attractive anymore and in my mind I believed that John wouldn't either. I focused on the big ugly indentation where my left breast had once been.

Sexually, in the past, my breasts had been a major player when it came to my love life. I loved nothing more than having my breasts sucked, touched and caressed. Now realising that sexually my breasts, or breast to me, was now a no go area, it would never be the same again; those experiences I had lost forever. The two of them worked in harmony with each other – left one, right one, a pair – just as God intended. That had all gone now; no more a pair. I hadn't thought that I would actually feel grief at losing my breast, but that is what I was experiencing. It wasn't just a breast; I now realised it was my sexuality, pleasure, attractiveness and intimacy. I felt robbed and cheated.

John entered our bedroom at that moment and, without thinking, I automatically covered my body, not wanting him to see my horrible disfigurement. Puzzled, he asked me what the matter was.

"My body is a mess now. A woman? That's a laugh. I don't look like one anymore and I definitely don't feel like one," I told him, as tears filled my eyes.

Instantly John casually walked towards me and, directly facing me, he lightly kissed my lips then said, "Roseann, the way your body is now is as beautiful as it was before your surgery. I love you and everything about you," he told me.

He then gently and slowly moved his head down my body, then simulated a kiss to my right breast as he said the words, "I love you". He then slowly and with the gentlest of movements placed his lips on where my left breast had once been, then again simulated a kiss, but this time said, "I miss you".

I could have cried with joy at his actions. You have no idea how wonderful he made me feel. Those few brief gestures made me feel almost whole again and any apprehension that I may have had at not wanting to share the sight of my disfigurement with anyone, not even my husband, disappeared. I realised then that he too felt the pain, the pain of what we had both lost, the pain of seeing how badly I had been affected by the change in my body and the pain of watching me struggle at times through what seemed like a neverending emotional rollercoaster. Knowing that John still loved me for me and not for what I once was; now that's what I call true love.

I had a two week period prior to the start of my chemotherapy treatment where I didn't have to attend hospital and it felt great. On one of those days I decided that I would walk down to the local petrol station not far from our house. I was so excited just thinking about being able to tell John what

Cancer No Not Me!

I had managed to do when he came home that day, given that I had not ventured over my doorstep without one of my family by my side. You see I was so terrified of someone bumping into me and also, truth be told, I had lost a lot of my confidence since losing my breast.

Usually one of my sisters or my mum and dad would spend a few hours with me each day whilst John was at work and that day was no different. My mum and dad had been and gone and it was after they had left that the idea of going out alone had came into my head. With it being around 2pm in the afternoon, I imagined there wouldn't be much chance of someone getting too close to me. After all, there were no children about as they would all be in school, plus the petrol station on most occasions was never really that busy. I was so proud of myself walking slowly down the street and, once there, pushed open the door of the shop adjacent to the petrol station. I felt a great sense of achievement. Given that I had nothing really in mind that I wanted to buy, I decided to browse through the magazines that were on display.

Whilst there, I noticed one of our neighbours just as he was about to leave the shop. Instinctively and with excitement I called across to him to say hello. However, on noticing me he seemed rather embarrassed and without saying a word he quickly left the shop. I was totally gutted. I just stood there wishing the ground would open and swallow me. How could he do that to me? Was he that stupid not to realise just how his actions would upset me? It wasn't as if I wanted to get into deep conversation; I had only said "Hello" and that was from a distance. In those few short seconds, he had successfully ruined everything; my confidence and the elation at my achievement. Panic overwhelmed me again as

Cancer No Not Me!

I just wanted to be back in the safety of my own home. It took so much effort trying to hold back my tears as I tried my best to hurry home. Once inside, I just sat alone and cried my eyes out.

It's strange how people tend to shy away from bad news, illness and the big C, never really knowing how best to handle it. Some find that the only way they can cope with this type of situation is to run in the opposite direction. Others are sympathetic and tell you they know exactly how you feel, although how can they, unless they too have been faced with the same illness? Maybe they say these things truly believing that their words will make you feel better.

All those involved with a cancer victim have been hit a heavy blow and all are devastated by the news; however none can truly understand how the other feels. They all want to be there 100% for the victim and yet the sufferer also wants to protect their family in whatever way possible. For example, I wanted so much to take my mother and father's pain away at having to cope with their child having a life threatening illness. Then there was my son Billy who wanted to alleviate my distress whilst in that cancer ward, instinctively going into protective mode by wanting to get on the telephone to find out what was going on in order to fix it. But none of us really truly knows how the other feels, or what they are going through.

I tried to imagine how my parents were feeling, but I could only really surmise, as I wasn't the one with a child who had cancer. I didn't have a clue how my son felt at having a mum with cancer. I knew he was devastated and in an instant would have taken my cancer himself if he could have, but deep down inside I could not see or contemplate just how much he was hurting. Looking at John my husband, although constantly supportive and dedicated in helping me get through this, he must have experienced thoughts of "Why me? Why us?" as well as low points and feelings of despair. How were my sisters coping?

Then there was me. I was very fortunate in the fact that I had so many people who loved me, but when it came to the actual cancer and the blows my body had already endured and still had to go through, I was alone. No one could see inside my head to truly understand how it felt to be the one with the cancer. Yes, they could try their best to understand, but believe me, unless you have been diagnosed with cancer yourself, you can only do your best by guessing. It's truly a conundrum of raw emotions for everyone involved.

As the days went by, I gradually grew stronger and overcame my encounter with my neighbour. However, what happened did adversely affect my desire to go outside on my own.

My pain, I am glad to say, had also reduced considerably and the horrendous tearing feeling in my chest that I had all too often experienced had completely disappeared. Feelings of tiredness continued to overwhelm me at times, but it was full steam ahead as with everyday I thanked God that I was still alive.

Feeling quite confident one day, I told John that I wanted to have a go at driving again. Excitedly I looked for the car key, desperate to sit behind the wheel. With the key now firmly in my hand, I made my way to the car with John following closely behind. Eagerly, I lowered myself into the driver's seat. I had it all planned. There was a small pillow positioned over the left side of my chest for protection both from the seat belt or any unexpected bumps in the road once I was in motion. I was all set for the off and was so pleased with myself once

I had turned the key in the car ignition. Hand firmly cupped around the top of the gear stick, I instinctively went to push it forward, but I couldn't do it. It was as if I had no power in my arm or shoulder. We have all heard the saying "Put your shoulder into it"; well my shoulder just wouldn't go.

My brain was sending signals telling me to move the gear stick, but the same signals didn't appear to be reaching my arm and shoulder. I must have tried about 10 times to move that bloody gear stick, but the more I tried the more frustrated I became. I was so angry with myself at not being able to do this simple task. Eventually I had to admit defeat and give up, which in turn only ignited floods of tears. Head down, I made my way back into the house feeling miserable. The whole experience was also quite frightening. I remember the intense fear I felt as I wondered if I would ever be able to drive a car again.

I only wished that someone involved in my care had taken the time to tell me that this might happen, given the type of surgery that I had had. I know it only seems like a little thing most probably not worth mentioning, but believe me it doesn't feel that trivial when it's happening to you. I'm sure that if I had been warned what to expect I would have had a better understanding as to why I was unable to perform this simple task. Anyway, you will be glad to know that the power did eventually return in both my arm and my shoulder, although it did take some time. I was so ecstatic the first time I successfully put my car into gear; I felt as though I had reached a major milestone in my quest to get back to the old me.

John and I had been in our local on a few occasions since the removal of my breast. Everyone that we knew there was very supportive and to some extent protective. There would always be someone there in an instant to make sure

I had a seat well away from any strangers and with plenty of room to ensure that there was no possibility of me being bumped. On some occasions I would stay for an hour and on other occasions only ten minutes; it all really depended on how I was feeling that particular day. The time that I stayed truthfully didn't matter; it was the fact that I was out there and not hiding away, something I could so easily have done after my encounter at our local petrol station. I was adamant that the forthcoming changes in my appearance would be accepted in a matter of fact way, just as it was happening, not as a, "Oh my God, did you see Roseann today; isn't she looking terrible?" which I believed would have happened if I had not ventured out regularly.

Some of the time though, the last thing I wanted to do was go out to our local, but given that this was one of the goals that I had set myself and because it was important to me that I was not looked upon as a hopeless case, I was determined to show the world I could do this. By remaining in one of the social circles that had been part of my life, I could draw strength from it.

Sometimes, whilst John and I were there, we would often meet up with the male friend that I had mentioned earlier who had won his own fight with cancer. More often than not, he sat with John and me, acting almost like a bodyguard at times. I think the fact that he had gone through so much of the treatment that lay ahead for me had something to do with it. He would constantly say to me, "Now if you don't have anyone to go with you to the clinic for your chemotherapy treatment, just give me a call." I always thought how nice it was of him to offer and if I had been someone who had little or no family, I know I would have most probably looked upon his gesture as a Godsend. Given the fact that I came from such a large family, however, that was never the case, although it still did not stop me from appreciating the offer.

I was lucky to have so much support from the people in our local; one of the barmaids had herself been previously diagnosed with breast cancer and on many occasions had been able to offer me valuable information and advice, when I was either worried about a lump or a bump, or scared of the unknown. It was through speaking with her that I found out that my impending radiotherapy treatment would not be painful, much to my relief.

There were also other local people who had also survived cancer; people to whom I had never paid much attention, but now it was as if I was becoming a member of an elite and sometimes secret group of people, all of whom had this enormous unseen bond of respect and understanding. I was touched by so many people that had either been through cancer themselves or who had a close family member fighting to win their battle against this awful disease. Sadly, I also heard of some who were unsuccessful in their fight.

Chapter Twelve

Chemotherapy: I'm Ready

It had arrived; the day of my first chemotherapy treatment and God was I nervous. I hadn't slept well the night before through worrying about what lay in front of me. An army of mostly negative thoughts filled my mind: Will I be violently sick whilst having my treatment? What about my hair? Will it fall out as soon as the chemotherapy drugs enter my body? Will I be plagued will constant vomiting? Will I be constantly tired and have no energy? What if, for some reason, they have to stop my treatment? Would that mean that nothing further could be done for me? What if my Hickman line became blocked and they couldn't get a vein? How would they then be able to get the chemotherapy into my system?

I needed to speak to Veronica, my chemotherapy nurse and have my questions answered. With that decision firmly in my mind, I began to make a list of all the questions that I wanted to ask her that day.

Arriving at the clinic with John by my side, I instantly handed my appointment card to the receptionist that I had met on my previous visit to the clinic. I was surprised by her instant recognition of me and how she spoke to me as if we had known each other for some time.

"Roseann, take a seat and I will let Veronica know that you have arrived," she said to me with a smile.

It was around 9.30am and John and I were the only two people in the waiting area of the clinic. As we waited, John began to talk, making lighthearted conversation with the odd joke thrown in.

"You might come out with a silhouette of radioactivity that will make you glow in the dark," he laughed.

To be honest, I think it was just his way of trying to help calm me down as I nervously shuffled my feet from side to side, not really knowing what to do or what to expect.

Scanning one of the walls, I was intrigued to see that it was totally covered by leaflets, some of which had big bold writing and highlighted help groups for people or families that were faced with cancer. I got to my feet and made my way to the wall for a closer look, finding it hard to believe that I had not noticed these on my last visit to the clinic. Glancing over other fact sheets, I found them full of information on many different types of cancer. There were even some that focused on the issue of secondary cancer. I was amazed by just how much information was contained on this one wall.

Veronica soon appeared and beckoned me to follow her into the treatment area of the clinic. My stomach was churning at this point. I tried to put on a brave smile, but deep down I wasn't coping that well at all. I remember thinking to myself that I didn't need the chemotherapy to induce sickness because I felt physically sick at just the thought of having it administered. Taking John's hand to make sure that he was coming with me, I got to my feet and walked in Veronica's direction.

I was glad that my appointment had been arranged for early morning, because I hoped I would be able to ask Veronica about all the things that had concerned me earlier without having other people around to hear what was being said.

"Veronica, there are a couple of questions that I wanted to ask you," I heard myself saying, almost in a trance like way.

Assuring me that she would try her best to answer all my questions, she also told me that if there were any that she could not answer, then she would do her utmost to find out, either through speaking to one of the oncologists or a fellow chemotherapy nurse. Her words momentarily helped me to relax a little. At least I could rid myself of some of the unnecessary mental torture I had been putting myself through.

"I just need a few minutes to get all the things together that I require in order to administer your treatment, then once we have everything up and running, we can go through the questions that you want to ask me," Veronica said.

Was having chemotherapy really that simple? I would have never imagined that this nurse would have been able to hold a conversation whilst my chemotherapy was being administered. I assumed the whole procedure would need her undivided attention and would be rather complicated. However, by the relaxed way in which she went through the motions of preparing all the things that she needed, it was clear that this was not the case. I watched her closely as she set up a drip stand and a trolley, on which she put a dressing pack and a few syringes. She also added a couple of small glass bottles filled with fluid, which I knew from having my Hickman line flushed contained sterile water. On the bottom shelf of the trolley, she had also placed a few small clear bags of fluid and two very large syringes containing a strange, reddish coloured substance. Looking at it more closely, it was apparent that this was the chemotherapy drug as it was covered in warning and hazardous signs.

"These are a Godsend; no trying to find veins, which can be a nightmare at times," Veronica voiced, as she looked directly at the two tubes that protruded from my body.

She then went through the process of flushing my line, before connecting it to one of the small plastic bags of clear fluid hanging from the drip stand positioned beside me.

"This is an anti-sickness drug," she explained.

Continuing, she told me that once this drug had passed from the bag and into my body, she would then link me up to the other bag for the same process to be repeated; that is, with a slight difference. This time the fluid would be saline. Once this drip had been set up and started, the chemotherapy drug would be injected into one of the tubes of my Hickman line and administered in conjunction with the saline drip.

I held my breath in anticipation, not knowing what to expect as Veronica proceeded to inject the first syringe of the chemotherapy drug into my line and through my bloodstream. Now all that was left to do was sit and wait whilst the remainder of the saline fluid gradually passed through my drip. That would be the completion of my first chemotherapy treatment. I'm glad to say that it was neither painful, nor caused any feelings of sickness. I was amazed.

"I'm all yours now, ready to answer any questions or queries you may have," Veronica said, as she took a seat beside John and me.

"I have a very and open and honest relationship with both the doctors and my breast care nurse involved in my care," I explained.

It was important to me that she knew I needed her answers to be honest; no avoiding or skimming over any subjects, even if she felt the answer to a question would upset me.

"That's fine by me; fire away," she said.

And I did, with non-stop questions about all the things that had being playing on my mind.

I must admit I was impressed by how Veronica handled the situation, relaxed and reassuring and definitely with a flare of confidence. She told me that as I was now aware, an anti-sickness preparation is given via a drip prior to the administration of my treatment.

"There is also an array of drugs that we can give you to take home that go hand in hand with the treatment you receive at the clinic to combat most of the sickness problems that patients may encounter," she added.

She then went on to answer my queries with regard to losing my hair, explaining that my impending baldness was really an individual thing.

"Some people lose their hair more quickly than others, although usually this will occur around 4–6 weeks into a person's treatment."

On asking her about what would happen should my Hickman line become blocked, she pointed out that as it merged into two lines there was a minimal chance of that happening.

"If one blocks, then we use the other," she explained.

This was something that had not crossed my mind, although after having it pointed out to me, I realised the answer to that question had been right in front of my face.

"Believe me Roseann, even if your two lines became blocked, we are experts in finding the smallest of veins, so don't let that worry you," Veronica assured.

During the rest of our conversation it was explained to me that I would most probably experience bouts of tiredness, but again that was an individual thing and depended on how my body responded to the type of treatment that was being given. Weight was also something that was important; this was because the dosage of the chemotherapy drug administered was determined by body weight. I was also intrigued to find out that my chemotherapy drug came from a different hospital; I had automatically assumed that it was prepared in the hospital where I received my treatment.

Veronica and I covered lots of ground that first day. I was told that with regard to my immune system, it would be approximately 10 days after my treatment that my white blood cell count would begin to drop and my body would become susceptible to infection. I was informed that it was also crucial that a patient's bloods are monitored on a regular basis, usually the week before a treatment is due, to ensure that the white blood count has returned to an acceptable level. Should this not be the case, then a blood transfusion would then be required.

It took a few hours that day before my treatment was complete, although I am glad to say that my worries about the initial administration of my treatment were really all for nothing. I had been neither up nor down during and after my chemotherapy treatment that day and left the clinic, doggy bag in hand, containing everything from anti-sickness drugs to oral antibiotics.

One thing that John, Billy and I had to consider was how we were going to tell my grandchildren that their gran would soon have no hair. They were only aged four and six and although very young would still have to be told. On their weekly visit to our house just after my first treatment, I decided to tell them. The way I approached it was by first starting a conversation with the girls on the subject of my illness and two operations. Both girls were well aware that their gran had been in hospital and wasn't very well, so off I went. You know Gran has not been that well and needed an operation? Well, so that I can get all better, I need to have lots and lots of medicine."

There they were, two little girls waiting to hear what their gran had to say next and all the while focusing on every word that came from my lips.

"The medicine I need," I went on, "will make me better, but might make me lose my hair for a while."

There, I had said it.

They both looked at me in astonishment, almost as if they expected me to tell them that I was only joking. However, my words were not followed by laughter and they both remained silent. Then out of the blue, Nicola the youngest spoke first.

"Gran, I don't want to see you with no hair on your head."

Now how could I answer that? What words would make her understand the importance of my treatment? None really. They were far too young. All I could do was explain to them that this was something that was going to happen, but that it was alright if they did not want to see me with no hair.

"You don't have to see Gran's bald head," I told Nicola. "I'm going to have a wig and if I am not wearing that I will put on a hat or a scarf," I reassured her.

To my surprise our conversation ended shortly after. It seemed the girls were quite happy once they had been reassured that they would not have to see their gran's bald head. The two of them then went on their merry way into the back garden and within a few moments I could hear their laughter as they played away, apparently unfazed by what had just been said. It's amazing how resilient children are.

My next port of call on the road that I faced was to visit a wig specialist in the centre of town. The appointment had been made by Veronica whilst I had been at the clinic for my first course of treatment. As far as I was aware, this was standard procedure. Apparently they felt it was best that patients choose their wig before they lose their hair; that way the wig fitter would have a better idea of what wig best suited the cancer patient's own head of hair.

I went with my mum and as we sat waiting to be attended to, I half heartedly joked with her about how I wouldn't mind if she wanted to borrow my wig on the days she could not be bothered to style and set her own hair. I must stress, however, that I do not think I would have been as jovial if I had lost my hair prior to my visit to the wig specialist.

A woman in her early 40s was responsible for assisting me in my search for my new head of hair. From talking to Veronica I knew that some patients take the opportunity to pick a wig in a style and colour that they had always wished their own hair had been, but I wasn't that brave. I was happy to let the woman get on with her job and before long we were down to three possible options. They all looked very similar really, but no matter what one happened to on my head, my mother would enthusiastically tell me that it was lovely. She was trying so hard to make sure I kept my spirits up. Love you mum! Anyway, we eventually opted for the one as near to my own head of hair as possible and after having it carefully packed by the assistant, we left the shop.

Once home, my poor wig was the centre of many jokes from my family, although I knew this was their way of trying to make light of my plight. Everyone in the family had a go at trying it on and then came the coaxing for me to do the same. When I did, they all made a point of emphasising just how much it suited me as well as stressing how real it looked, although from my point of view I didn't think so. It's funny how the person who has to wear it for real and those who don't have totally different views on the subject.

I was certainly impressed by the quality of this false head of hair, but knew that I would never feel comfortable wearing it and imagined if I did, everyone would have instantly known that it was a wig and not my own hair. I can understand that not all recipients in need of a wig felt as I did, knowing only too well how this item for many is a blessing.

I was surprised at just how well my body seemed to be coping with the strong chemotherapy drugs that had been administered. Yes, I had felt sick, but it wasn't intolerable and the anti-sickness drugs seemed to work a treat. I had also been given an antibiotic liquid that I had to put into my mouth daily via a dropper. That wasn't that bad either and I remember thinking, "If this is as bad as it gets, then I could sail through the whole thing easily."

By the tenth day after my first chemotherapy treatment, I was well aware that this would be around the time when the efficiency of my immune system would start to reduce dramatically. That was why it was imperative that I took the oral medication to help my body fight off any possible infection that might try to invade my mouth. I had been told that the mouth is usually the first place to be hit by infection, because of the amount of bacteria we all have floating about in there. With the breakdown of the immune system, it's almost like an open invitation to all the little germs in your mouth to have a big party. Apparently it doesn't take long for them to spread throughout your mouth once they have successfully broken down the minimal defence system that you now have. Not only does the chemotherapy attack any cancerous cells, it also attacks the healthy cells of your body as well. It's a matter of weighing up the benefits against the pitfalls really and in my case the possible benefits far outweighed the disadvantages.

It's strange how much one's priorities and needs change. I tried hard to set myself small achievable goals to help keep me sane and positive, yet on the other hand, a goal that I had set prior to my diagnosis no longer interested me. That goal was to receive a diamond ring from John on my 40th birthday, which was also the day of our wedding anniversary. It was something we had planned prior to my illness, a special token of the love we shared for each other. I had so looked forward to that day, the day I would be able to wear something so very precious with pride, but now my dreams of that moment had now been replaced with feelings of dread and sadness at possibly never experiencing that moment. It was almost as if this ring would end up as a symbol of my death.

Although I tried most of the time to stay positive, a nagging doubt that I would not win my battle for life would still periodically emerge; a feeling that I now know never leaves you when faced with cancer. Feeling as I did at that time, I truly believed that there would be no worth in something that I would most probably never have the chance to enjoy. The whole point had been to be able to look at this symbol of love as the years went by and to recall the excitement and joy we felt when buying it and of what it represented. But now, with my diagnosis of my cancer, I felt robbed of these dreams.

Would I ever get to be a silver-haired old lady? The reality was that I didn't think I would. I told John that I no longer wanted the diamond ring I had so excitedly looked forward to receiving. It would just be a ring if I didn't have the years that were meant to go with it.

"It's not about time, Roseann; it's about love," John had told me, but if I wasn't there to give or receive that love, there was no point. It saddens me that I felt this way.

About a week after my second course of chemotherapy treatment, my impending hair loss was not far away. I recalled Veronica's words of how hair loss would probably begin 4–6 weeks into a patient's treatment and I was now at the 6 week mark. It started slowly coming out when I rinsed my hair after washing it. Not a great amount, but nevertheless I knew that from that moment on it was only a matter of time before all the hair on my head would be gone. As the days passed by, I would notice my hair regularly lodged in my hair brush. Strangely, I had also begun to experience sensitivity around my hair follicles and if I happened to be outside on a windy day, I would experience mild pain and sensitivity as gusts of air flowed through my hair. Even running my fingers through my hair caused pain, almost like having a slight toothache. It was a persistent pain that was becoming more frequent and was something that I had mentioned to Veronica one day at the clinic. She looked at me puzzled and said she had never heard anyone mention these symptoms. It just shows you how right they are when they say the way your body copes with the treatment is very much an individual thing. I never mentioned these symptoms to anyone else. To tell you the truth, I felt rather silly when Veronica seemed not to understand what I was talking about.

That was it, I decided one Saturday afternoon as John, Billy and I sat watching television. I was going to get John to help me wash my hair and if my hair loss was more apparent, then this would be the day that I would ask John to shave my head. There was no way I was going to wait until I had big bald patches all over my head, personally feeling that this would look a lot worse than having no hair at all.

As John washed my hair, I could not believe how sensitive my scalp had become since its last wash. If I had any previous doubts about what I was about to do, then they truly went out the window as I gritted my teeth whilst John rinsed my hair and my scalp tingled. That was it; the remainder of my hair was coming off. I think John and Billy only half believed that I would go ahead with it, that is until I had set up the hair clippers we had used for cutting John's hair.

As I sat on a stool at the ready, I must admit I was so very close to changing my mind. I had dreaded the thought of having no hair and here I was telling John to shave it off. There was no going back now, as John drew the razor over the top of my head. Watching my hair fall to the floor, I was surprised to find that instead of crying I had in fact started to find the whole situation rather amusing, especially when as John had finished one side of my head and handed the razor to Billy, who then proceeded to shave the other half. All together we laughed as we shared what must have been one of the most intimate and private family experiences that I had ever had; the two most important men in my life sharing such a dramatic moment.

That was not the end of the hair cutting session. After my head had been completely shaven, John and Billy both had their heads shaved as well. First John and I shaved Billy's head as we giggled away to ourselves and then Billy and I shaved John's head. After we had finished, all we could do was stand there laughing at the sight of each other, all bald coots together.

My husband and my son most certainly made the whole experience of losing my hair so much easier for me by sacrificing their own hair. I don't think they could have ever realised just how loved they had made me feel, or how much they had boosted my self-esteem by doing such a selfless act.

It's amazing just how cold you feel when you have no hair on your head and how susceptible you become to the slightest of drafts. I was glad that I had already begun collecting different hats and scarves for the arrival of that day. I sat with a mirror in front of me trying all the different ways in which I could wear a scarf. I had it tied under my chin, then behind my head and tied at the base of my skull. I even tried it up the way the land girls wore theirs during the war. That gave John and Billy a good laugh I must admit. I'm sure the two of them had thought I was losing the plot and that my hair loss had gone to my head. Ha! Ha! I even tried wearing a scarf and then a baseball cap on top of it. I must admit I was impressed by how much wearing them both together actually masked the fact that I was bald. It was then that I knew for sure that this was the option for me, rather than a wig.

In a way I was rather relieved that the apprehension and stress at the thought of my hair loss had been lifted. Excitedly I telephoned all my sisters, my mum and dad and John's mum. Now all I had to do was to wait in anticipation at how my granddaughters would react now that I was bald.

Running into the house, both girls then stopped dead in their tracks and gazed at the scarf covering my head.

"Are you bald now Gran?" Nicola asked, as Rebecca looked on with her mouth wide open.

On telling her that I was, both stood silent. You could almost feel the intensity of their thought processes. Nicola could contain herself no more.

Gran, is all the hair on your head shaved off?" she asked.

"Yes," I told her.

"So you have no hair under your scarf at all?"

I tried hard not to laugh as Nicola's inquisitiveness increased.

"Do you want to see it?" I asked both girls, as they stood with their eyes transfixed to my head.

"I don't want to see your bald head Gran," Nicola said.

Reassuringly I told both girls that it was alright to feel that way and they did not have to worry because I would always make sure that I wore a hat or a scarf when they came to visit.

"But what about your wig?" Nicola piped up.

The girls had known that I was going to have a wig because this was something that we had explained to them when we had initially brought up the subject of me losing my hair.

"Oh, I have it upstairs, but I didn't want to wear it. Would you like to see it, or try in on?" I asked them both.

Excitedly they both nodded, then watched as I made my way out of the lounge towards my bedroom. Walking back into the living room, I tried hard to contain my amusement at the sight of my two granddaughters sitting side by side, silently waiting to see their gran's new head of hair. Taking time to look at my wig, they both tried it on; first Nicola and then Rebecca. Billy, John and I all laughed merrily as we watched the girls play with the wig.

"Gran, can I see under your scarf?" Nicola asked out of the blue.

"Sure," I told her.

With that, I slightly lifted up the front part of my scarf to reveal a small part of my bald head.

"Can we see all of your head?" Nicola bravely asked, as poor Rebecca looked on apprehensively, not knowing quite what to do. I slowly lifted my headscarf off.

"There! That's Gran with no hair," I quipped lightheartedly.

The girls then told me that they were no longer frightened at the thought of me with no hair and quite happily ran into the back garden to play as like any other day.

The whole issue of my baldness had been accepted by the girls as just another part of my illness. I'm sure my son must have been so proud of his girls at the way they had handled the whole situation. I knew I definitely felt pride. I am so fortunate to have not only two beautiful granddaughters, but two very special ones.

My whole life now seemed as if it was no longer mine. All I ever seemed to do was attend clinics or be seen by medical professionals. I was grateful to every one of them for their skills and expertise in assisting me in my fight against cancer, but that did not stop me from becoming fed up at times with the intensity of my treatment.

I was attending the chemotherapy clinic 2–3 times over a 4-week period and my district nurse Isabell visited me at home 2–3 times weekly. I also had regular visits to my own GP, appointments at both the breast and oncology clinics and a few other appointments at the cancer ward because of flu like symptoms and a high temperature. In addition, I was attending a clinic held by Jean to have my wound monitored and also to have fittings for a more lifelike breast prosthesis. To cap it all, I had also received my first appointment to attend a physiotherapist at the hospital who specialised in dealing with arm problems associated with extensive chest wall, breast and lymphatic surgery.

I was also beginning to suffer more from the side effects of the chemotherapy treatment. I was now experiencing more problems with sickness and had been given a stronger anti-sickness drug to help alleviate this. Although they did help, I still felt slightly nauseated most of the time. The antibiotic mouth drops were also beginning to make me sick at even the thought of having to put them in my mouth, but thankfully these were replaced by the drug in pastel form, which made it so much easier for me to tolerate.

Horrendous constipation now plagued me and my muscles and bones ached so badly at times that I felt it almost impossible to put one foot in front of the other. When feeling this way, I felt like just collapsing on the spot where I happened to be standing. Strangely though, at other times I would feel that although I was exhausted my body just would not shut down and no sooner had I sat down than I would find that I would have to stand up and be doing things. It became a standing joke in our family (pun not intended). They would comment that I must be taking speed again. Obviously I wasn't, but it was their way of making light of the fact that I sometimes seemed to want to move at 100 miles per hour. Being fatigued one minute and wanting to run around like Roger Rabbit the next was contributing to the fact that I was now suffering from depression.

Night times were hard for me. At times I would be desperate to sleep, but couldn't and more often than not would spend countless hours alone downstairs with only my thoughts for company – and sometimes my thoughts were not very good company at all. I sometimes sat in tears at not knowing what to do to ease my physical pain or my emotional turmoil. I would sometimes feel so frightened and at these times would be in desperate need of John's company and reassurance. But with all the care and assistance he was giving me during the day, how could I expect him to also be there for me through the night? If he had known half of what I was going through, he would have been there for me 24/7, regardless of his own health, But how could I do that to him? In my eyes, he was already pushing himself way beyond the boundaries of emotional and physical pressure. Therefore, most nights I would slowly and gently ease myself out of bed and creep downstairs, to once again spend hours of solitude with only morbid thoughts as my companion.

On other occasions when I would experience really very low points where I felt I could take no more, I would go to the kitchen, regardless of time, and begin to grill either bacon or sausages. Once ready, I would slowly make my way upstairs and kneel at John's side of the bed, then whisper that I had made him breakfast, even if it was only 5am. I think the breakfast was really my way of saying to John, "Sorry for getting you up, but I can no longer face being alone."

One day I had a really strange experience. My youngest sister had taken me to yet another one of my appointments at the chemotherapy clinic and on that particular day I was not feeling that good. I was feeling very downhearted and was finding it hard even to cope with the everyday things that we all have going on in our lives. Everything seemed to be taking such a long time; getting to the hospital, finding a parking space, the walk from the car to the clinic and so on.

The relief I felt on returning home that day was phenomenal to say the least. On entering the house, my sister automatically walked straight into the kitchen and put on the kettle while I stood in the hallway. Lifting my head, I looked to the stairs that lead to my bedroom. However, on this occasion they were now no longer just stairs to me; they looked like a bloody great mountain and felt like one too as I pulled myself slowly onto each stair. On reaching my bedroom, I just collapsed on the bed, thankful at being home. Struggling to remove my jacket, I gave up and just burst into a flood of tears. I just felt I could take no more as I rolled myself into a ball and just lay there alone on my bed crying. All the while, my sister was downstairs in the kitchen oblivious to what was happening upstairs.

As I lay there, the most relaxing feeling washed over me and I accepted that I was ready to die. It was as if the desire to fight my cancer had been punched right out of me and I did not want to struggle anymore. Strangely, as I came to terms with that fact, I experienced this amazing feeling of release. No more did I have the feelings of panic that I could possibly lose my fight for life and have to leave my family; a thought that would have horrified me before. I just felt so very tired and wanted to go to sleep and never wake up.

It gave my young sister such a fright that day when on entering my bedroom to see if I was alright, she found me lying there voicing how I could no longer go on and wanted to die. I must have put her through emotional hell as she tried endlessly to show me all the reasons for living. By the time she had finished, it was hard to determine who was the most exhausted – me or her.

I am glad to say she succeeded and with her help I got through that day, although looking back I can now understand how acceptance to impending death can overwhelm a person and, through my experience, I can easily understand the wishes of a gravely ill person to be left to sleep.

I have often wondered through my own experience of the passing of a close relative, watching how calmly they appeared to be when faced with death, if all who pass from this earth knowing that they are dying experience a feeling of acceptance and conclusion of their existence.

Meeting my physiotherapist for the first time was an experience and a half. On seeing her, I nearly hot tailed it back out of the physiotherapy department. She had called out my name in a very matronly voice and as I walked in her direction she then went on to inform me that her name was Marie Becks, emphasising Mrs Becks, before telling me that she was one of the senior physiotherapists in the department.

"Follow me Mrs Gallagher."

"Roseann," I corrected her, to which she responded that she preferred to use titles and surnames rather than be on first name terms with her patients.

"Oh God," I thought initially, "what have got myself into?

However, I needn't have worried. After a few more appointments with her to have intense therapy on my left arm in the hope of regaining further movement and power, she soon got fed up with me constantly telling her to call me by my first name, as I did when referring to her. In the end, she relented and we then both addressed each other by our first names.

It was funny, but as we became more familiar with each other, we did in fact end up in a very informal relationship, totally different to the one that I originally thought we would have. To be honest, I thought I would have ended up hating her, but that was not the case. Instead I grew to have a tremendous amount of respect for her, as she did for me. She was a true professional and an amazing physiotherapist.

Before meeting Marie, I must admit that my vision of physiotherapists was that they really weren't worth the bother and I had tagged them as hopeless. It was not until I worked with Marie that I realised just how much work these people do and also how they can regain and improve the movement of a limb.

This woman was marvellous. She knew exactly all the problems that I was experiencing with my arm and showed total dedication in my treatment. She also ended up becoming a confidante like Isabell, someone to whom I could turn to if needed. She also seemed to instantly sense when I felt low and would take time to find out what was making me feel that way. She would then, in a non-judgemental way, offer simple but effective solutions to my problems. In the end, she always had a knack of making me feel things weren't that bad after I had spoken to her and before I knew it I would be feeling a whole lot better.

One day, when I was feeling particularly ghastly, she once again restored my faith in my ability to go on and continue fighting my battle with cancer.

The day prior to attending my appointment, John and I had been to our local pub with one of my sisters and her husband. After sitting in the bar for a while, we all decided to make our way upstairs to the lounge. I was so pleased when I arrived there to find that four of the pensioners that I would sit with on occasions were playing dominoes. Sitting with my family, I could contain myself no longer. I was desperate to play dominoes as well, so off I went to the other side of the lounge, leaving John engrossed in conversation with my sister and her husband.

The day went well and I was truly in good spirits by the time both John and I arrived home. Excitedly, I told him of the laughs that I had shared that day with the men that I had been sitting with. John smiled, but seemed a bit offhand and at first I thought that maybe he was disgruntled that I had left him with my sister and brother-in-law. However, on asking him, he told me he wasn't and that he was happy that I had enjoyed my day.

Later that evening John still appeared rather quiet and whenever I asked him what was wrong, he would reply that he was just tired. Sometime later he was still the same and I pushed him to tell me what was troubling him. I went on and on and wouldn't let up; it wasn't like him to act in this way and it worried me that he looked so sad.

Eventually, John told me that whilst sitting with my sister she had made the comment about how sick she was of hearing about cancer, something that truly shocked me. I couldn't understand how she could make that statement and pushed John to tell me his reply to her comment.

"I told her she didn't have a clue what she was talking about as she wasn't living, as we both were, with cancer looming over our lives 24 hours a day."

On seeing Marie the following day, I burst into tears as I told her what had happened. I just found it so hard to believe that my sister could have let me down in this way. Marie, as always, was totally empathetic and offered her theory. She took the time to explain that in her experience she had found that people whose lives has been touched with cancer can act in the strangest of ways.

"Some family members become very protective of the person with cancer, sometimes to the stage of almost smothering their loved one. Others become very angry with the world and those of us who are in it, or are jealous of the person with cancer because of the attention they are receiving and others can act totally out of character due to the immense pressure they find themselves under," she said.

Putting it that way, who knows why my sister said what she did. I know she would be horrified if she knew how much her words had affected John and me. For this reason, to this day, I have never mentioned any of this to her.

On another visit to see Marie, I had ventured alone to the hospital, although the realisation of just how dependant I had become on others had hit me like a hard slap in the face, as I struggled to travel by bus alone. It was a silly thing to do and I realise that now, but I was eternally grateful once again to Marie for her support and reassurance.

I left the physiotherapy department still knackered from my journey that day, but at least with an air of confidence in my abilities. I could have so easily have got a taxi for my return journey home, but instead decided to slowly walk to the bus stop to clear my thoughts. Once there, I sat on a seat at the bus shelter going over in my head just how much Marie had been there for me. Before I knew it and from where I don't know, words started coming into my head about the way I felt about her. Let me share the words I wrote.

An Earth Angel

You have so many qualities,
I thought you had to know.
You're a special kind of person,
That has helped my life to grow.

From a weak and tired woman,
I strove to get on track.
To that individual person,
Not so long ago way back.

You have been a little Godsend,
A special kind of link,
That has brought me back so many times
When I was on the brink.

Cancer No Not Me!

I have felt that I can't cope at times
And thought of giving up,
But you have made me understand,
My faults and cheered me up.

These special words are just for you,
So you will understand
That sometimes every one of us
Needs a helping hand.

So whenever you are feeling down,
And wonder why you're here,
Just take the time to contemplate
The things that are so dear.
You know that life can't fault us,
For being what we are
And you my special Marie,
Are a guiding star.

You bring such hope and pleasure
To all the folk you treat
And without you there beside us,
We would surely feel defeat.

So protect your lovely healing hands,
For they have work to do
For the countless many people
Who are blessed to come to you.

by R.P Gallagher

To Marie my Physiotherapist. June 2000

On my next visit to see Marie, I took the poem with me, which I had typed and framed. Leaving the physiotherapy department that day, I handed her a bag that contained the poem, telling her to open it once I had gone. I only hope she liked it.

Breast reconstruction was a topic that I had discussed with both my surgeon and also with Veronica my chemotherapy nurse and, to be honest, I felt that it was taken for granted that this would be something that I would want, given my age. However, I was in two minds about the whole thing and really didn't know if I could have tolerated such surgery. If this was something that I had wanted, it was explained to me that I would have had to wait until all of my chemotherapy and radiotherapy treatments had been completed. My strength and recovery from my treatments was also something that would have to be considered. I knew from conversations that I had when being treated by different doctors, that this was an important fact to be considered before any form of surgery would even be contemplated. However, I did not know if this was something I really wanted to do; if I had chosen to go through with this kind of surgery, it would most probably have been for all the wrong reasons. In other words, I would not be doing it for myself, but for John. Not that he had given me the slightest inkling that he thought I should have the surgery; if anything, he had felt that I had been through enough and advised me against it.

I have met a few women who have gone through this procedure and, like everything, it had its benefits and drawbacks. The benefits would be that for some of these women it would make them feel a whole person once again and would aid in restoring their feminine side that they felt had been taken away from them. I could understand that this was very definitely important to those women who felt that way.

One woman who had gone through the surgery had the muscle from her back almost detached, then swung around to be used as her reconstructed breast, which I am glad to tell you was obviously done under a general anaesthetic. She had told me during one of our conversations in the chemotherapy clinic that she had hastily had it done at the same time as her mastectomy, although in hindsight she wished she had waited until after her treatment before having this procedure done. Her reason for this was that the time that it had taken for her to heal and had caused her chemotherapy treatment to be put back. The medical team dealing with her case knew that if they had started her treatment before she had healed properly, then as her immune system began to break down, her own natural healing processes would be greatly affected and healing would take much longer.

Some other drawbacks I was told about were very strange, if not funny. This same woman had also told me that every time she scratched her reconstructed breast, she would experience the sensation not in her chest as you would assume, but on her back from where the muscle to make the reconstructed breast had been taken. We both found that rather amusing, although she was told this was only a temporary setback and would rectify itself once her brain had compensated for the change.

Another area commonly used in the reconstruction of a breast is the stomach, although I had not spoken to anyone that had undergone this type of procedure, so knew little about it.

Since breasts are presently the topic of discussion, this I feel would be an appropriate time to tell you in more detail about breast prostheses. Some are made of soft fibres like the type I was given initially after my mastectomy and others are made of a jelly like substance that feels very much like a real breast. The benefit of the ones made of the jelly substance is that they have the weight of a real breast. This is a property that breast prostheses made up of soft fibres do not have and this can be a drawback in that gravity obviously pulls your breasts down. The soft fibrous type of prosthesis has no weight, so you can find when wearing this type that you have one breast up higher in your chest wall than the other. No matter how many ways you try to adjust your bra to compensate for this imbalance, the result remains the same; one up and one down.

The problems this causes can be a right pain in the butt. You don't want to leave the house, because you have difficulty getting your clothes to sit properly. It would really upset me at times when I was faced with this dilemma, although I'm glad to say that I no longer have this problem, given that I have a snug, jelly lifelike breast that is very effective at doing its job.

Chapter Thirteen

It's Good to Laugh and be Blessed by Friends

I maintained close links with our local pub and visited it on a regular basis, even when I had great difficulty trying to muster up the energy to go. On these occasions I would make John take me down, even when I could see in his eyes that he obviously thought it was a bad idea, either because he felt I was too ill to go, or because he could see that I was in pain. I'm sure I worried the hell out of him. We would often laugh at the effort it took for me to get there, only to enter the bar, take a seat and then ten minutes later say that I couldn't do it and wanted to go home.

Another thing we would laugh about was how the thought of Vodka and Coke, my usual aperitif, would make me feel physically sick and how we would both scan every drink behind the bar in search of one that did not invoke nausea. When we actually picked one, I would take a sip and then hand it to John, telling him I could not drink it. At least I tried!

Other days I would be on great form. I would even manage to play a few games of dominoes with the local pensioners who frequented the bar. I was so proud of myself if I successfully stayed in our local for an hour; anything over that was an achievement in its own right. Sharing these times in the bar opened so many doors for me. It gave me the opportunity to make new friends, some of whom remain so very dear to me even to this day. It also helped in boosting my self-esteem. At times I was even able to share a joke or a laugh with some of our locals. I remember one day when I was feeling particularly well and took myself up to the bar to buy a round of drinks for the company that John and I were with; I was wearing a baseball cap that day to mask my baldness. Anyway, whilst standing at the bar a man slightly older than I jokingly went to remove my cap saying, "Are you bald underneath that?" Instinctively I put my hand on top of my head in order to ensure my cap stayed on whilst at the same time replying, "Yes I am."

Talk about wishing the ground would open up and swallow me. This poor guy's face was a picture as he struggled for words and I returned to the company I was with, leaving him standing there totally embarrassed. Thereafter, every time I crossed paths with this guy, he would apologise profusely for his actions. He even went as far as to tell me that if I ever needed a blood transfusion, he would be only too happy to oblige. Funnily enough, after that we got on like a house on fire and he is now a very dear friend of ours. To this day, I still pull his leg about the time he nearly removed my baseball cap.

I have to tell you about Heather my next door neighbour and the day she practically walked me into the morgue; yes, the morgue. On that particular day, Heather was my escort to yet another hospital appointment. She always stepped in to help if a member of my family was unable to go to the hospital with me. I was well into my chemotherapy treatment and more often than not I looked and felt ill. After being seen at the oncology clinic that day, we both took a slow walk down the link corridor that took you from the new part of the hospital directly into the old part. We talked about how great it would be when I had finished all of my treatments, as well as everything and nothing really. We were so engrossed in conversation.

Now to put you in the picture, the morgue of the hospital was situated just off the middle of the link corridor and to the right, but the exit that we usually took in order to get to the car park was also situated off and to the right, but it was further down the corridor and beyond the sign that said "Morgue". Anyway, before I knew it, Heather was taking a right turn, not to the exit that we usually took, but the one that would have led us to the morgue. Realising that this was what Heather had done, I turned to her said nonchalantly, "Heather, I am not ready to go to the morgue yet."

Well you should have seen her face; she was totally horrified at what she had done and was bright red with embarrassment. I just could not stop laughing at how she had reacted and in the end the two of us I am sure nearly wet ourselves, we laughed that much. It was truly a very memorable moment that I still kid her about to this day; somehow I don't think I will ever let her forget it. I still get a kick out of saying to her if the both of us are in conversation with another person, "Heather tell them about the day you took me to the morgue." Even the reaction on the face of the person we happen to be talking to at the time is a picture. It's as if they are trying to work out whether or not they have heard correctly. When given the full story, they too get just as good a laugh out of it as we do.

Heather was married to Ian and they had a daughter called Diane and a son called Ross. Both she and her family were a great support to John and me. Nothing was ever too much trouble for them and I am sure any of them would have run from here to hell and back for us.

I felt great one day at being able to help Heather for a change. She was stuck on Wednesdays for someone to keep an eye on Ross after he had returned from school, as everyone in her family worked later than usual on that day, so I offered to watch him. It was only for a matter of a few hours and to be honest I was really looking forward to being able to spend the time with Ross. I had always felt more like an aunt to him than just the next door neighbour.

John had happened to be out one particular Wednesday, so on that occasion it would be just Ross and I to keep each other company. More often than not though, it was more Ross looking after me than me looking after Ross, a role I must say that he took very seriously.

Ross was around 11 years of age at this time, so watching over an adult for a child of that age must have felt like a huge responsibility. More often than not, I would spend most of the time that Ross was in my house lying on the sofa, whilst he would busily play with some sort of electronic game plugged into the television. He was an angel who always made sure that the game he happened to be playing was not too loud to become an annoyance to me. Periodically he would lift his head up from whatever game he happened to be playing at the time and asked if I was alright, or whether I needed anything, which to me was priceless.

The time past quickly that day and before I knew it Ross was getting his school satchel and was telling me that it was time for him to go home.

That day, like all the other days since losing my hair, I had one of my patterned scarves over my head and tied at the nape of my neck. It was very rarely that I would be seen without one, unless in the company of very close family members.

As Ross walked to the door, he instantly opened his arms and wrapped them tightly round my body, then planted a kiss on my cheek, taking me totally by surprise. Sadly, my reaction was to instantly pull away from him. Given that I am a very tactile person, this is something that I wouldn't have normally done. A cuddle or a kiss to someone was usually my way of saying goodbye. However, given the way I looked – no hair and gaunt as hell – I thought I might have scared the living daylights out of poor Ross or, even worse, feared he would pull away from me in disgust. In a half joking voice I told him, "Oh Ross, I did not kiss you because I thought you would not have wanted me with my bald head and all," trying to make a joke of the situation. But joviality turned to pride as he turned to me and said that he loved me and to him I was beautiful. I felt like a million dollars and to this day his words still fill me up with emotion every time I recall them.

Another funny story involving Heather was the time we were coming back from yet another chemotherapy clinic appointment. Again, I didn't feel that grand and could not wait to get home. As we made our way into the street in the direction of Heather's car, I was physically aware of how heavily I was leaning on her as she took my arm. As always, we were chatting non-stop. As we approached the traffic lights to cross the road, I suddenly became aware of a work lorry from the corner of my eye. There must have been at least six workmen in the cabin at the time. Just as the lorry passed us, the driver of the vehicle loudly sounded his horn. Lifting my head and interrupting Heather mid sentence, I said, "It's me they were looking at" in my most pathetic voice. Heather immediately got the gist of what I was talking about and burst into laughter. Yes, I might have been feeling like shit that day, but that did not stop me from being quick off the mark with a little quirk. Not bad for a bald headed chemotherapy patient wouldn't you say?

I also have to tell you about the time John and I were sitting in our local when one of the regulars walked through the door; on entering the pub, he instantly recognised John and sat beside us. He wasn't someone that I knew, but the minute he saw me the first words out of his mouth were, "You look like a pirate with that scarf on." People within earshot just looked on in amazement. On receiving an explanation from John as to why I was wearing a bandana, this chap put his hand over his heart and said, "Oh big man, I am so sorry; I would have never offended you or your lovely wife for the world." Turning to me he became rather emotional as he told me how sorry he was at saying what he did. Poor soul; I think he had originally said it to make me laugh, but instead he nearly had me in tears, not because he had upset me by his words, but because of the way he had genuinely been so remorseful for his actions.

Chapter Fourteen

Let's Start Round Two

I had now successfully fully completed my Doxorubicin chemotherapy treatment and the day of my first course of the combination of three different types of chemotherapy had arrived. My sister Iris had come with me that day. The clinic was certainly becoming a familiar place to all of my family, as well as Heather next door. As both Iris and I chatted away, Veronica had already prepared her trolley and started my treatment. I was at the stage where I was just about to be connected to the usual saline solution that was given to coincide with my chemotherapy.

"Well Veronica, that's me now on my second lap of treatment," I said, rather proudly.

Veronica smiled and said something like, "Good for you," and then went back to administering my treatment.

To tell you the truth, Veronica and I had never really hit it off, not in the way that I had with my district nurse and physiotherapist. I don't know why, because I had tried hard to develop our relationship into a more relaxed one, but was unsuccessful. Don't get me wrong; we had never had cross words and when attending my appointments we were always polite to one another, but we just didn't seem to click. After administering my new chemotherapy treatment, Veronica then left us to get back to our discussion, which couldn't have been that interesting because I cannot remember what it was we were actually talking about that day.

Cancer No Not Me!

What I do remember, however, was the sudden feeling of numbness I began to experience down the right side of my face, initially scaring the life out of me as my thought processes tried to make sense of what was happening. I remember thinking to myself, "Is this what a stroke feels like?" My heart pounded at the possibility that this was what I was experiencing. Panicking, I grasped at my sister's arm and told her of the numbness in my face, terrified that if I did not get the words out quickly I would soon be unable to speak. God was I frightened.

Iris instantly got to her feet and raced to find Veronica to inform her that something was terribly wrong. On returning with Veronica, my sister looked on anxiously as I quickly tried to explain to my chemotherapy nurse about the numbness, terrified that at any moment I could be struck down with the inability to converse. After listening to what I had to say, Veronica then casually informed me that what I was experiencing a side effect associated with the combination of chemotherapy drugs. She didn't appear in the least bit concerned by what had just happened, nor by the fact that I was upset.

I could literally see the anger rise within my sister at my nurse's explanation, because she had not taken the time to tell me what to expect and was even more annoyed that Veronica appeared not to care and had simply disappeared back to her duties. It took all my powers of persuasion to stop her from having a rather heated word with Veronica.

From that day forward, I kept any contact I had with Veronica to the minimum. "Good morning; how are you?" was the extent of the clinical relationship that I had with her.

A few weeks later on a return visit to the clinic for the usual check-ups prior to my next course of treatment, I was surprised to meet one of my father's old friends. Knowing that we could not ignore the fact that we had seen him, and given that it was apparent that my mother couldn't wait to go over and speak to this man, I reluctantly made my way to the vacant seat beside him. The last thing I wanted to do was become involved in a full blown conversation about why both my mother and I were at the clinic. When I think about it now, one must have been stupid not to realise why, given the fact I clearly looked unwell and was wearing a bandana.

I scanned the clinic to see if I could recognise the person he had come with that day, automatically assuming that he had come with a sick relative. Surprisingly though, I didn't see anyone that looked familiar. Not saying anything other than an initial "Hello", I took a seat and left any further conversation in the hands of my mother who loved nothing more than a good blether. I listened to the two of them talking of past times and of how they both had children that were married with families of their own. I remember thinking to myself, "Wait for it, Roseann; the next topic of conversation will be about you having cancer," to be followed by the usual platitude of, "I'm so sorry to hear that". However, this was not to be. Instead, I was the one who looked totally surprised as this man told my mother how he too had been diagnosed with breast cancer. That was the last thing I had expected to hear.

It turned out that this man had been diagnosed some years previously and had for a few years been cancer free. However, his cancer had now returned and he too was a patient of the clinic. Suddenly, I was now the one keen to have a conversation and before long we were in deep discussion about the forms of treatment that we were having and of all the side effects we had encountered. I couldn't believe how quickly the day passed and before I knew it we were telling each other to take care and saying our goodbyes.

Instead of a chance meeting turning into what I thought would be a dreaded encounter, meeting this man was truly an uplifting experience for me. We were able to share so much in the short period of time that we were together, as well as boost each other's morale no end.

On my visits to the clinic thereafter, I always looked out for him, but our paths never crossed again. It was not until the completion of my treatment and a chance meeting with his son, that I discovered that he had sadly lost his battle with cancer and had died about a year after my meeting him that day at the clinic.

So many people's stories touched my life. One that I found so sad and which almost brought me to tears was my encounter with a young girl who was only seventeen. She had fallen pregnant and had hidden this fact from her mother. It wasn't until she was only weeks away from giving birth that her mother realised the truth and took her daughter to see a doctor. What happened next must have shattered their lives; a routine blood test had shown that this young girl had Leukaemia.

When I first meet this young girl, she was by then a mother and would often bring her baby with her to the clinic when having her treatment. I and all the other patients would smile at the innocent laughter and actions of this baby who unknowingly brought a ray of sunshine into the lives of all at the clinic. The love this girl had for her child just spilled from every pore in her body. I so admired her for the way in which she coped with her situation. I thought a lot about that girl and often wondered how life could be so cruel.

Her story was published in our local paper in the hope of finding a successful bone marrow donor, although sadly I never found out if she was successful; she just seemed to disappear into the background without a trace.

On another visit to the clinic, I bumped into one of the three women with breast cancer that I had met whilst in hospital. She was the woman that I had mentioned before with the young daughter and a long history of breast cancer in her family. It was good to see her in high spirits and I was so pleased for her when she told me that she also had shown no signs of a relapse. She did tell me, however, that the oldest women of the three had detected a lump in her neck, which had turned out to be cancerous. I felt so sorry at hearing of this woman's plight, knowing only too well how easily it could have been me. With regard to the third lady – the one that found it so hard to accept her diagnosis – I was told that although she remained cancer free, she was apparently very depressed and had found it hard to cope with the chemotherapy treatments.

My body seemed to be coping with my new treatment of the chemotherapy combination regime, much to my relief. I could even say that the sickness had diminished considerably. No longer did I dread the thought of trying to eat, only to find that when I did I would be plagued with feelings of nausea. Sometimes, even the thought of food induced vomiting, so the fact that this had subsided boosted my morale no end.

I felt so elated at having successfully finished my last chemotherapy regime and the months of treatments that I felt I would never conquer now seemed achievable. I was even able to sleep much better, which made a great difference to me. The periodic feelings of wanting to rush around frantically remained, but I could cope with that. To be honest, after experiencing the need to go at a million miles an hour, I would slump down exhausted, but would feel a great sense of achievement at having been productive. Whether I had managed to run a vacuum cleaner over our lounge, or wash a few dishes, I would be so proud at what I had done and would brim from ear to ear at having been helpful to John in some way, rather a hindrance, even though John said I was not.

I had crossed a major milestone in my quest to beat cancer and was now well on my way through the second treatment programme.

Chapter Fifteen

Benefits, Bills and the People We Meet

I found my own experience of trying to access sickness benefits an absolute nightmare. On applying for a benefit known as Disability Living Allowance, I was faced with all sorts of hassles, which is the last thing someone with a terminal illness needs. I would often get so upset by the masses of bureaucratic paperwork that had to be completed. It is a scandal the amount of forms that have to be filled in and the countless questions that have to be answered. Then, to add insult to injury, you are asked to tell them on the forms how you are when you are at your worst. I found this ludicrous. Surely the fact that the person applying for the benefit has been through major surgery and is receiving a long course of arduous chemotherapy treatments speaks for itself?

Not only does the person have to endure extreme stress when trying to complete the said forms, they have then to wait approximately 3 months or longer before being told whether their application has been successful, which only adds to the existing pressure.

I know from my own experience how desperate I felt at having to wait 3 whole months for the outcome of my application. The worry of whether or not John and I would be able to keep our head above water was a great burden. We desperately needed some sort of financial aid, but any time we tried to access our wonderful benefits' system, we were constantly told that we were not entitled to any form of assistance; that is, with the exception of Incapacity Benefit, which sadly wasn't a great deal of help.

I was not even entitled to free dental or eye treatment, something I found appalling given that my chemotherapy treatments had affected both my eyes and my teeth.

It was always for John and I, as like many people I'm sure, a Catch–22 situation, in that we were one of the many on the border line, neither entitled to income support or aid with our council tax, because John worked. It just wasn't fair. John and I were not people who lived beyond our means, or idly refused to work. We were a couple who both worked damn hard and had based our lifestyle on the incomes we received. Not for a minute did we imagine that one of us would be struck down with an illness that would affect our ability to work. Yes, we knew that there would be times when one of us would be off sick from work due to mild illnesses such as flu or a chest infection, but never had we envisaged a situation where one of us would no longer be entitled to sick pay from our employer, due to long term sickness. Sadly, this was now the case. I had now run out of sick pay entitlement from my employer and found that instead of having a good monthly income, I only had a small state sickness benefit. Things were truly not looking that good for us with regard to our finances.

Even approaching our mortgage broker to ask if we could suspend our payments for a few mouths was a waste of time. My broker was very sympathetic to my circumstances, but with regard to easing our financial burdens, I was told that our mortgage would automatically fall into arrears if we did not keep up with our repayments. It wasn't as if I was asking for something for nothing. I had only wanted a few mouths of grace to ease some of the pressure. The last thing I needed to be told was that our mortgage would go into arrears.

One way that you could access the benefit known as Disability Living Allowance was under what was known as Special Rules. What this meant was that an application under this category required a section of the form to be completed by a doctor. By doing so meant that the doctor was basically saying that it was not expected that the person who was ill would live longer than 6 months. It was only in these circumstances that a person's application for benefit would then be hurried through the system.

In my opinion, this is just another way of gate keeping in that some doctors can be reluctant at times to make such statements. The fact that in some cases were the patient does not wish to be told they are dying also means that Special Rules are not applied, on the basis that it would cause that person great distress to find that Special Rules actually mean they are unlikely to survive.

I must stress that although I am sure many cases do get accepted under this category, more often than not this is when the person is practically at death's door.

With regard to my application for Disability Living Allowance, I was told that a doctor who represented the benefits agency would be visiting me at home to assess whether or not I was entitled to receive this benefit. On the day that he arrived to see me, my youngest sister Debbie was in the house with me. On introducing himself, the doctor then asked me to tell him the problems that I been experiencing with my health. It was staring him in the face! I looked terrible, I was undergoing chemotherapy, fatigue overwhelmed me and I ached from head to toe; the list was endless.

I gave him my medical history since being diagnosed with cancer and told him of all the health problems that I was experiencing, which was then followed by a request from the doctor to examine me. On telling him that he could, he then proceeded to ask me to take his hands in mine and squeeze it as hard as I could. This I had to do with both my right and then my left hand. After asking me to first stand then sit down, he then took a seat next to me. Scanning my body with his eyes he stated, "That's a very nice suntan you have Mrs Gallagher; have you been somewhere nice?" I could hardly believe my ears. Taken aback and by now rather angry, I quickly spat out the words, "No doctor, this is not a suntan you see; this is in fact a side effect of my treatment."

I went on to tell this stupid man that the chemotherapy drugs that I was being given changed the pigmentation of the skin. "You cheeky bastard; where do they get you people?" I thought to myself.

The next test he then gave me was an eye test. I was asked to stand at the side of my bed whilst he walked into the hallway; he then proceeded to hold up an eye test card and asked me to read from it. To be honest, by this time I was beginning to wonder if he had lost the plot.

After he had completed all his tests, he then informed me that I would be told if my application for this benefit had been successful by post, in about another 4 weeks. Wait for it; the best is yet to come. On his way out of my house, in the presence of my sister, he said, "Mrs Gallagher, you have to try and keep positive. I mean I have had patients that have come to me on countless occasions saying they just knew they had cancer and inevitably these people did in fact end up with this terrible illness. Can you see what I am trying to say? In other words, it is important that you try to remain positive in the belief that you will beat your cancer." He proceeded to tell me how sorry he was to hear of my diagnosis, then left, leaving us both totally dumbfounded by his words.

He was right about one thing though; I did hear from the benefits agency four weeks later via post. They informed me that my application for Disability Living Allowance had been rejected. Where is the justice in this world? I am glad to say that in the end, through the intervention of my local councillor, the decision with regard to my case was eventually overturned. So please let me stress to all of you out there, if ever applying for any form of benefit for either yourself or for a member of your family, do not struggle to complete those complex and stress provoking forms. Instead, get either your own doctor or the social services department in your area to refer you to someone who is trained in this field to complete these forms on your behalf.

Hospital transport is another thing that we know little about. We tend not to think that it is a resource that we are entitled to, or are able to utilise, should we need it. You do not have to take up the services of an ambulance. Taxis, hospital cars and patient transport ambulances used specifically to transport patients to and from appointments are now widely available. The hospital you are attending or your own doctor can arrange this form of transport for you. Those who find themselves too sick to travel by public transport and have no family or friends that can drive them to and from their appointments can benefit from this form of service.

I was one of the lucky people in that I had family, friends and neighbours that I could rely on and therefore did not require this service. But there are many people out there that do so desperately need it and if you happen to be one of them, I hope this information has helped you.

Now here is something that people don't give much thought to until it is upon them and that is telephone bills. Before you know, it they have escalated at an alarming rate. You might say that it doesn't matter, but it's another outgoing that you don't need as every penny begins to count. Another financial strain is the last thing you need on top of what you already have to deal with, but sadly it is cruel fact of life. It's not just the phone bills, but all the other little things, like prescriptions for instance. It's hard to believe, but because of the financial burdens John and I began to experience, I began to find it difficult to pay for all the prescriptions that I needed. If it weren't for my mum and dad buying me a yearly prescription certificate, I think I would have opted for making do with what I had.

In my opinion this is another area where the government or health services let people down, as I learned from my own experience. We were not quite in the income bracket to be eligible for free prescriptions, but neither were we well off. Like many people, we were in the in-between bracket.

Other outgoings you don't consider are hospital parking fees. On occasions, I found that I could be in a clinic for anything up to three hours and all the while the parking meter still ticks away. John would constantly have to keep returning to our car to feed more money into the meter.

Heating costs is another area. Because I was now in the house all day, my heating would be on at times when it would normally have been off. Nobody thinks to tell you about all these little stumbling blocks that become a financial problem when added together.

Sad to say, another financial worry that looms over your head is funeral costs. We are all aware that a funeral is not cheap these days and it terrified me to think that if I were to die, there would be no immediate money that John could just put his hands on to cover the costs. In the long run he would be entitled to our life insurance, but that was tied up with our mortgage. In other words, if I were to die then the house would be paid off by the life policies in my name. He would also most likely be entitled to something from my work, but with regard to a pension, this was something I had always meant to do, but like many had put it off for one reason or another, not thinking for a minute that I would be hit by a life threatening illness. I never suspected that I would have ever had to face any of these issues at the age of 38, or obviously I would have fully prepared for it.

John was now on long term sick leave like me; everything had got too much for him and his doctor had given him a sick line for stress. Although this had helped in alleviating some of the stress that John had been under, it had sadly also put added strain on our purse strings. Part of John's salary was based on a weekly bonus and given that he was not at work to earn that bonus meant that he would lose about a third of his normal take home pay.

It's really quite frightening when you are faced with having to cope with everything associated with the cancer and on top of that face the possibility that realistically you could end up losing everything you have worked so hard to acquire, through no fault of you own.

Would we get through this? I hoped so.

Chapter Sixteen

He Was Nice and They were Awful

Although I rarely ventured out, when I did I seemed to have a whole new outlook, refusing to pass someone who had made an impression in my life, thanking them for their assistance or acknowledging them with either a "Hello" or "Take care".

I had been out with John for a run in the car and was desperate to blow off the cobwebs around my gills. On our way home, I asked John to stop at our local co-op store as we had run short of milk. As John stopped the car, he automatically opened the car door on his side with the intention of going into the shop. Quickly I stopped him. "I'll go in and get the milk," I said. John asked if I was sure that I would be able to manage. "Yes," I reassured him. So on opening the car door on my side and with a gentle push from John to help me out of the car, I made my way to the entrance of the store.

I felt slightly uncomfortable at still having no hair, although I did have a scarf over my head. I could feel the stares from another woman who, like myself, was in to make a purchase. She was anything but subtle as she looked at me with a stare that was so intense that I could almost feel it penetrate my back as I walked past her. I really hated it when people did that. You expect children to look at you because they are inquisitive as to why you have no hair, but when adults do it, it makes you wonder where they get their manners from. Anyway, I in turn stared back at this woman, determined not to let her attitude spoil what must have been my first visit to this store since being diagnosed with cancer.

Slowly I made my way to the refrigerator that contained the milk, picked up the carton that I wanted and walked in the direction of the cash desk. As I stood waiting for my turn to pay, I could feel the energy drain from my body. Not for a minute would I have expected that such a small task could exhaust me so much. I felt as if my turn at the cashier's desk was never going to come. I was thankful that John was still sitting in the car, oblivious to how difficult I was finding the simple task of buying milk.

Suddenly, I was approached by the security guard of the store, whom I initially assumed was going to speak to one of the other customers, but I was wrong.

"Are you all right? Would you like a glass of water madam," he asked me.

Surprised by his thoughtfulness, something that is in short supply these days, I thanked him for his kindness but declined his offer of water. "How considerate," I thought, as I felt a smile come to my face. This man's actions made all the effort of purchasing the milk worthwhile. As I left the store, I smiled in his direction as another gesture of thanks, then made my way to our car.

"How did you get on?" John asked, as I slumped into my seat exhausted. Telling him that the whole experience had taken such an effort, I added it had been worth it, if only for the experience of feeling the satisfaction it had given me at being able to do something on my own.

As a further gesture of thanks to the security guard, I later found out what his name was and made a point of writing to the store's head office commending this man's professionalism, observations skills and kindness, highlighting that I felt he was an asset to the store in which he worked.

Little things do really mean a lot; this chap proved it, as I hope I did by submitting my letter.

Issy came over to my house as she did nearly every other morning to see if I needed anything. On telling her that I didn't, she said her goodbyes, telling me she had so much to do that day before going to her work that evening. She worked in the local biscuit factory not far from where we lived. Not long after, John put on the kettle to make both of us a cup of tea, but just as he was about to set up our cups, he discovered that we had run out of sugar.

"I'll nip across to Issy's and borrow some," I told him, glad at the thought of having the chance to get out of house for a bit of fresh air. It was great having a sister living so close; I never had to worry about running out of anything because nine times out of ten Issy would have it and vice versa.

On my way back from my sister's house, sugar in hand, I couldn't help but notice two boys of around 16 years of age who appeared to be posting something through the letterbox of one of our neighbours. As usual, I had been wearing one of my many headscarves. Just as I walked past these boys, I could hear them talking to each other, but could not make out what they were saying. I carried on walking, uninterested. As I reached the drive at the front of our house, out from the mouth of one of the boys came a shout loud of, "Is that a wig on your head?" followed by loud laughter from the both of them. Never for a moment did I suspect that they would jeer me as I went by. I instantly became embarrassed and upset by it. As I turned to look at them, it was obvious the boys were deriving great pleasure from making fun of me. Now I found myself rushing in a panic to get to the front door of my house, desperate to escape their teasing.

On entering our front doorway, John immediately noticed that I was upset and asked me what the matter was, as by this time tears dripped down my face. When I told him what the boys had said, he marched right out of our front door without saying another word. Within a matter of seconds he had caught up with the boys and was towering over them as I watched from our front window.

"Do you think that you were being funny?" he blasted at these two boys, the smiles now gone from their faces.

John told them if they wanted to make fun of anyone then they were to make fun of him. It was one of the very few occasions that I ever saw John so angry. Looking rather ashamed, the boys mumbled that they were sorry and that they hadn't meant to upset me. At that John turned and began to walk back to the house.

"They have been delivering that free local paper," John said, as he began to search for our telephone directory. "I'm contacting their head office; they are not getting away with upsetting you in that way," he told me.

Just at that moment, one of the newspapers hit the floor of our hallway. John nearly scared the living daylights out of the woman who had put it through our letterbox, as he frantically swung our front door open. The poor woman was frozen to the spot. John was in a rage and I was right behind him to make sure he didn't do something he would later regret. The woman just stood there with her mouth open as John asked her if she was in charge of the boys that had also been delivering the paper. When the woman informed him she was, John told her what had happened.

This poor woman was mortified and explained to us that the two boys were in fact her son and his friend.

"Rest assured, I will certainly deal with this matter," she told us both. "I just can't understand it; I do a lot of charity work for people who have cancer and my son is aware of that fact."

Apologising, she assured us that she would speak to both boys.

"And believe me I will," she said, as she then walked away, very embarrassed by the whole incident.

Sometimes I find it so hard to make sense of how some people can be so kind and obliging whilst others can be so hard and cruel.

Chapter Seventeen

I'm a Poet and I Didn't Know It

As the weather improved, I would often sit in our front garden and write poems. I had well and truly got the bug since writing that one for Marie. It was important to me that I put into words how I felt. Please let me share the rest of my poems with you.

A Husband's Love

One day I heard some awful news,
I thought, "I cannot cope,"
But you have brought me back to life
And given me true hope.

You listen to my fears each day,
Although you have your own,
But put them to the side most times,
So I won't be alone.

You've seen the massive change in me,
Both in body and in mind,
But you have never said one word,
That I can say is unkind.

True love I only share with you;
I've known from the start
And to you, my darling husband,
I give to you my heart.

by R.P. Gallagher

To John, the husband in a million. 21 July 2000.

My Child

Mothers are a special thing,
They bring such joy and everything.
They cannot be explained at times,
But understand that you are mine.

I live to bring you love and joy,
Throughout your life, both man and boy,
So please believe in what I say,
There never will be any day
That I don't think of you and say,
That God has blessed me every day,
Since giving birth to you.

You've made me proud that I'm your mum,
A blessing that has truly come,
From you my only darling son;
A man now you've become.

I love you more than words can say
And think of you throughout the day.
So when you think of me each day,
Just think of all the words I say,
'Cos then I'll know you're with me too
And feel the love I share with you.

by R.P. Gallagher

To Billy, my darling son. 20 July 2000.

Cancer No Not Me!

My Strength

You run around and never stop,
You keep on going until you drop.
The pain, you look it in the eye
And dare yourself not to cry.

Your ailments we will never see,
There deep within you, like the core in a tree.
Exceptional you surely are,
My added strength, my guiding star.

My aches, my pains, my days of doubt;
Without you I can't do without.
I love you more than words can say
And will be there for you in any way.

So when you feel you cannot cope,
Just think of me and you'll gain hope.
You see I'm just as strong as you
And there for you when you need me too.

by R.P. Gallagher

To my sister Iris. 20th June 2000.

Respect: A Man Called Bill

When lying sick in 42,
You hear so many things,
But in this ward that I was in,
The patients constantly sing.

A song, oh no, I do not hear,
But praise for yet another,
An extraordinary individual,
Who sounds just like a brother.

I'd never met this man they spoke of,
But truly was intrigued
And when I finally met him,
Charmed I was indeed.

When meeting him I understood,
The praise they gave to him,
For pouring from his very soul,
Was kindness to the brim.

He has a wondrous talent,
When caring for the ill;
Making us forget how sick we are,
Is a very special skill.

He brings such relaxation,
To ease away our fears
And encourage echoes of laughter
Instead of the sound of tears.

He looks beyond our illnesses,
Just like a guiding star
And chooses to see us not as now,
But as whom we really are.

by R.P Gallagher

To Bill, Chemotherapy Nurse. July 2000.

I don't profess to be a poet, but found I had to share my words with you.

Chapter Eighteen

Back to the Grind

Being told you have cancer gives you a whole new perspective on life. I have shared so many beautiful moments with my family that I know would have passed by as just another day if it hadn't been for the fact that I had the knowledge that I could die sooner than I had anticipated. It was as if a part of my heart and soul that I would have never opened to the outside world, had suddenly the need to be heard.

I wanted to tell my son with a passion how much I loved him, how when he came into this world and after being placed on my chest by the nurse, he had lifted his head, eyes wide open as if to say, "I'm here". I wanted to write words that expressed my emotions for another. I needed my mum and dad to know that I was still their little girl who loved them very, very much. I had to tell John that our marriage and life together had made me whole and with regard to my sisters, I wanted to embrace them, physically and emotionally.

Quality time had a whole new meaning to me; things that I had once found mundane were now precious. I had a second chance to look at my life; it was almost as if I had mentally detached from my body and was looking from the outside in. I took more time to see all the wonderful things in the world that I had previously taken for granted.

Having to face death is almost like being shown something that is unseen by people who have not had to face this awful dilemma. It is like a vision of life itself.

I was now two thirds of the way through my combination chemotherapy treatment and I'm glad to say the side effects of my treatment were very mild compared to the ones that I experienced whilst having the Doxorubicin. The terrible sickness I had experienced in the past still remained under control and I was now even able to go back to using a milder form of anti-sickness drug. This was a relief, given that these types of drugs are also a bugger for causing terrible constipation, something that can be an absolute nightmare, especially when you're not feeling yourself in the first place. It is so uncomfortable not being able to go to the toilet. I would get so fed up at the time that I spent in the loo hoping that just maybe this might be the moment when I would be able to go, only to find that yet again nothing happened. On the occasions that I had successfully been to the toilet, given that it was often a very rare event, I almost wanted to shout out to the world! Believe me, the feeling of relief at being able to "go" on a regular basis had certainly lifted my spirits.

With regard to feelings of fatigue and then my moments of frenzied activity, these still remained, but strangely enough I was actually coping rather well with these side effects and had begun to accept them as normal.

Nerve-ending pain a result of my radical surgery was another kettle of fish. It felt as though every nerve in that part of my body was electrified. Even just brushing against something would be a nightmare. I would constantly be like a cat on a hot tin roof if anyone came close to me; there wasn't a day that went by without me having to grit my teeth because of the pain.

Losing my eyelashes was traumatic for me; I would even go so far to say that it was one of the hardest things to accept through all my surgery and treatments. Whilst going through some chemotherapy treatments, hair loss as you are aware is a common side effect. I had eventually resigned myself to that fact and I thought that I was coping well. What I never gave a thought to was that it was not just your scalp hair that you lost, but also every other hair on your body. It just hadn't occurred to me until I experienced it firsthand.

Losing my body hair had not affected me the way that losing my eyelashes did; it was as if I had lost yet another part of my femininity. No matter how bad I looked, I could always put on a little mascara and still feel at least slightly feminine. But this all disappeared gradually with every lash that I lost. It's hard to put into words just how it felt to no longer be able to put on a little mascara. It was as if a safe place had been stolen from me. No longer could I hide behind my lashes, which made me feel that I was telling the world with pride, "Look at me; I'm coping".

Being unable to do this was certainly a great blow to my self-confidence. People might say that a little thing like that does not matter if you have your life, but believe me it does. People noticed when I had made the effort to put on mascara and would often comment on how this small act had made a difference to the way I looked, in a complimentary way. Unless you have experienced it yourself, you have no idea how much it means to someone in such a position to be complimented in this way. At times it made me feel as though I was walking on air, proud in the fact that I could still receive a compliment with regard to my appearance.

Given the fact that the chemotherapy regime that I was presently receiving was a 6-month course made me feel at times that I would never get to the end; it just seemed to go on and on. Yes, I did feel more able to cope and, yes, I did have fewer side effects, but the fact that I still had a long way to go before reaching the end of not only this treatment but also the course of radiotherapy that was to follow, often got me down. I felt like a specimen in a jar that was constantly brought down from its shelf to be once again examined or prodded.

There were now more good days in my life than bad, but when those bad days appeared, it felt as though an interminable black cloud had positioned itself directly above my head and would not be budged. No matter how hard I tried to pick myself up, doom and gloom would overpower me. I would get so pig sick of having to endure the countless appointments to all the different clinics and departments that were so much a part of my life. On occasions I am certain that I mentally talked myself into a depressive state. I would allow myself to dwell on the vast changes in my life, or open my inner self to the morbid thoughts from the past that once haunted me: "Am I going to die? Is this struggle through treatments all for nothing?"

When this happened, I would experience long sullen moments where I did not want to talk to anyone. To tell you the truth, it got to the stage where the only way I could cope was to go to my bed and pull my duvet over my head in the hope of blocking out not only the world, but my feelings of misery. Any level of noise on these days became almost unbearable and I would find myself literally at the point of madness if not in the sanctuary of my peaceful bedroom.

When recalling these times of blackness and mixed emotions, I can now logically say that it was most likely a very bad case of depression that made me feel this way. But when these experiences are actually happening, logic is the last thing that comes into the equation. Only now can I look back and say that it was alright for me to feel the way I did, or that I would not have been human if I hadn't experienced these feelings, given the situation I found myself in. But again, it doesn't feel that way; instead you have an overwhelming feeling of guilt at letting yourself get to the point of insanity, which is just how I felt at times.

On a lighter note, I have to tell you about the one and only time I ever wore my wig, which I am pleased to tell you, was one of my better days. Issy was constantly on at me about how real it looked and that no one would ever know that it wasn't my real hair,

"You should wear it," she would say.

In the end, after eventually getting so fed up at her going on about it, I thought, "Ok, I will go out with it on", really just to keep her happy more than anything.

As I had an up and coming appointment at the chemotherapy clinic, I thought this would be the opportune time to choose as the day to christen my wig. As soon as I had stepped out of the house to get into our car with John, I felt instantly uncomfortable and on our way to the hospital I must have asked him dozens of times if this thing I had on my head looked as if it were real. I really don't know how he managed to keep his head! I must have driven John to near madness that day.

Sitting in the front passenger seat of our car, I felt as if all the people in the other cars that passed us by were looking directly at me with this wig on my head. The more I looked, the more I believed that everyone was looking at me whilst thinking to themselves, "God, is that a wig she has on her head?"

Getting out of the car on our arrival at the hospital didn't make me feel any happier about my new headdress. If anything, I felt worse and walking from the car to the clinic was a nightmare for me. I walked with my head constantly down and only once did I find the courage to look up, although when I did I instantly felt as if I was the object of everyone's stares, so quickly returned my eyes to the ground.

By the time John and I had arrived at the clinic, I could take no more; it had to come off, even if it was only to maintain my own sanity. I was so relieved that I had the sense to put one of my bandanas into my bag before leaving the house. I couldn't wait to get into the patient's toilet within the clinic, as John looked on amused.

I felt nothing but total relief as I pulled this thing off of my head, scratching my scalp, as it was by now itchy as hell and sighing with relief as I popped the wig into my bag. "Never again," I thought as I manoeuvred my head scarf into position.

Relief was written all over my face as I walked towards John.

"Feel better now?" he asked me.

"No John, I feel bloody marvellous," I told him.

Now I know that wigs and hair pieces can be of great benefit to some people, but I was not one of them. I felt too self conscious when wearing one and the discomfort was terrible. My poor scalp was roasting as the temperature soared under this hairpiece. I remember thinking to myself, "Anybody who can go through even an hour, let alone a day, with something like that on their head deserves a medal".

John had been shopping, leaving me alone in the house. I was exhausted and decided to rest rather than push myself to the limit that day. On hearing the telephone ring, I instantly picked up the receiver expecting John to be on the other end of the phone checking that everything was alright. I was so surprised when answering the phone to find that instead of John's voice on the other end it was the voice of a man who was unfamiliar to me.

"Can I speak to Roseann Gallagher?" the man instantly asked.

"Speaking," I told the caller, wondering who this person was and why he had wanted to talk to me.

It turned out that this man was a professor at the Caledonian University, explaining further that he had just found an application I had submitted (a few months prior to my diagnosis) to do a degree in social sciences. Going on, he told me that he had no explanation as to how my application had managed to be filed wrongly, but now that he had looked over it, was telephoning to offer me a place at the university. I could hardly believe my ears; I had assumed that by not hearing from the university shortly after submitting my application, that I just hadn't been good enough to make the grade. I listened on as an enormous feeling of pride and achievement washed over me.

"I would like to offer you a place in our September intake," he told me.

Thanking this man for taking the time to contact me, I told him how I would be unable to except his offer, explaining my reasons. On saying that he was very sorry to hear that I had been ill, he then continued by saying that he would be more than happy to hold an unconditional place for me in their February intake the following year. I was totally overwhelmed at being given this news, so much so that after talking to this man in great depth, I accepted his offer, with a promise that I would to keep in touch. After putting down the telephone, I almost wanted to run rings around my living room and was filled to the brim with excitement. I just couldn't wait for John to come home so that I could tell him my news.

John was so over the moon for me and listened eagerly as I went over the conversation that I had shared with this professor. The following day I was still excited as I got dressed to go to the chemotherapy clinic for my next course of my treatment.

Sitting in the clinic watching Veronica prepare my treatment, I could no longer contain myself. I had to share my news.

"You will never guess what happened to me yesterday," I told her excitedly. Not waiting for her to answer, I continued, "I was offered a place at university."

I waited for her reply. Talk about putting a damper on things.

"Well you know what it's like these days; bums on seats – that's all these places are really interested in," Veronica replied.

"You bitch," I thought, "How could you be so cruel?"

There was no way I was going to let Veronica get away with her horrid words.

"No, Veronica," I told her, "it's not just a matter of bums on seats; those bums have to have the qualifications to enable them to sit on those seats in the first place," I fumed.

Veronica knew I had been angered by her response to my news and chose not to say another word on the subject.

Iris my sister had been with me that day and like myself could not understand how nasty Veronica had been.

"Never mind; you put her in her place," Iris told me.

I never shared another word with Veronica about what was happening in my life after that incident.

It makes you think doesn't it? I had applied for a place at university and if I had been given that place at the time that I had applied, I would have inevitably had to stop due to my cancer diagnosis. I always thought that strange; it was almost as if some other force was watching over me and held back my application in some way because it knew beforehand that I would be struck by cancer. Maybe our loved ones do watch over us.

Strangely enough, after all my excitement, I declined my place at university. After giving it a great deal of thought, I felt that before being diagnosed with cancer I had to prove to myself that I could achieve a degree. However, after my diagnosis, my whole outlook on life had changed and I knew in my heart that I no longer needed to prove to myself I had the capability to gain a degree. I knew I had. Another reason was that realistically I did not know how much time I had left on this earth. Given that fact, I chose not to tie myself up in four years of studies, opting instead to spend every precious moment with the people I loved.

Given the realisation that my body would never be the same again, I started to re-evaluate what clothes would now best compliment my new body. I cleared out all of my low cut tops and dresses from my wardrobe and instead of looking at it as being almost like a bereavement, I accepted the fact that this kind of clothing was no longer for me. Instead I told myself that I would now opt for attractive, but high collared tops, something that had a positive impact in rekindling my femininity.

Yes, I still had to live with feelings of not being the whole person that I used to be, but now I had begun to re-educate myself in ways of how to dress in order to mask my body and its shape, which also worked wonders in improving my own self-esteem. No longer would I be the timed and self conscious individual that this illness had made me, or that person that had to live with long and baggy clothing that dreaded being looked at by others. I had regained some of the old me and was ready to show the world.

During a consultation with one of the doctors at the chemotherapy clinic, I had asked if it would be alright for me to go on a short holiday. I was over the moon when he told me that I could, but then became instantly flat when he followed on with, "but I would advise that you choose somewhere in Scotland." I had been thinking more along the lines of going down south to see my younger sister Janet, but there you go. I suppose it was better than not having a holiday at all.

On arriving back from the clinic, I could hardly believe how excited I had begun to get at the prospect of getting away from it all; it was almost like experiencing a great release. John and I would be free to do what we wanted and all without having to think about doctors, nurses, clinics and neverending treatments. I was so happy. I couldn't wait to tell Issy, knowing that as her husband worked all over Scotland, she would be full of helpful advice on where best to go.

"Oh Roseann, Pitlochry is a beautiful place; a quaint little village with lots of lovely scenery and I know a lovely hotel there you would just adore," she told me.

My sister explained that both she and my brother-in-law had once stayed at a rather upmarket hotel that had a swimming pool. She didn't have to tell me anymore. I instantly knew that this place would be ideal given that John just adored swimming. The fact that there was actually a pool on the premises meant that I wouldn't have to worry or feel guilty about John being stuck for things to pass his time during the day on the occasions that I needed to go for a lie down.

Any doubts that I may have had at the cost of this hotel were quickly washed away as I told myself that this was really just what John and I needed. All that remained for me to do was to check that John was happy with the choice. Once I had told him all the details, he too was as excited as I.

After making our booking via telephone for the following Saturday to Tuesday, I rushed over to Issy's house to tell her our plans.

On the day we were meant to leave for Pitlochry, I awoke feeling really exhausted and with no energy at all. I couldn't believe it; after counting down the days with excitement, I now felt that the thought of leaving my house was the last thing I wanted to do. John tried everything that day to persuade me otherwise, but I would not budge. There was no way I could have travelled all the way to Pitlochry that day.

"We can leave on Sunday instead," I told John, as I wrapped my arms around him and gave him a great big cuddle as a way of trying to make up for spoiling our plans. "I'll contact the hotel and explain that we will be arriving on the Sunday instead; it's only a slight change and we can make up the day at the other end," I told John, as guilt began to eat away at me.

The hotel was only too happy to assist and obligingly made changes to our reservation at no added cost.

The weather was fantastic that weekend and I'm glad to say my health wasn't too bad either. My sister was right; Pitlochry was truly a beautiful place and John and I enjoyed every minute that we spent there. With no pressures looming over

Cancer No Not Me!

our heads, we went for slow walks and visited all the local places of interest. The place even had its very own castle with huge grounds filled with Highland cattle. There was also a river where you could sit on its banks and watch the salmon leap. It was so peaceful and relaxing just sitting there watching the fish periodically jump out of the water, with no thoughts of hospitals racing around my head. We had an absolutely fantastic four days away. Although totally exhausting for me, the exhilaration at getting away was well worth it.

With regard to our accommodation, the hotel was rather la-di-da, not somewhere we would have normally picked to stay, but we enjoyed it all the same. It was really quite amusing watching the mannerism of some of the other guests, not to mention listening to their conversations. Some quite clearly thought that they were definitely the bee's knees. I could hardly believe it when one guest actually snapped his fingers in order to attract the attention of a waiter. How ignorant can you get? John wasn't that impressed by this pompous guy's manners either.

We would always make a point of leaving a reasonable tip for the staff, not because we had cash to throw about, but because we could see just how hard the staff worked and wanted to show our appreciation for their excellent service. We knew only too well, given that John had done this type of work in his youth, that as the staff were young seasonal workers, many of them foreign, they were probably paid very poorly.

The staff were so very obliging to us and constantly went out of their way to look after us. They knew we were different from the usual clientele that visited the hotel and I think they were just glad that someone actually had taken the time to respect and appreciate the work they did. One of them even made our day by stopping in the centre of town to excitedly show us their tongue piercing, which I must say amused us no end. By the end of our holiday, John and I were both in high spirits and were once again ready to face anything that life chose to throw at us.

On our way home, John suggested that we drop in on my mother to let her know that we had arrived home safe and sound.

"Alright," I said, rather puzzled by John's suggestion as I assumed he would have been exhausted after our long drive back and desperate to go straight home.

"Hi, mum, we're back," I shouted as I went through the door to my mother's house.

Looking at her face as she appeared from the kitchen, I remember thinking how my mother always looked so worried these days. My cancer had certainly taken its toll on her.

"Are you coming up to ours for a while?" John piped up from behind me, to which my mother instantly replied "Yes."

Before I knew it, they were both hurrying me back into the car. I thought their actions odd and to tell you the truth wondered what all the rush was about. However, not wanting to say anything to John about it in front of my mother, I just went with the flow.

I thought it even stranger when my front door key would not turn in the lock.

"This is certainly not turning out to be my day," I thought.

"Issy has probably dropped the latch on the door by mistake. Don't worry, I have the side door key," John said.

"Thank God," I thought to myself, not relishing the fact that my mother and I could be left on the doorstep as John went in search of my sister.

Cancer No Not Me!

Opening the door that lead from my kitchen to our lounge, I found it hard to believe my eyes as I stared open mouthed at the complete change in the lounge and dining area. My sister Issy stood proudly in the centre of the room. Tears ran down my cheeks as I took in the bright fresh décor and a brand new carpet.

"Do you like it daughter?" my mother asked, as tears also filled her eyes.

"Oh, it's beautiful," I said, as I went to first hug my mother then my sister.

"Now you know why I wouldn't decorate the living room for you when you asked me," John told me.

I felt instantly guilty for the way I had nagged at John a few weeks previously. I had given him a really hard time about wanting our living room decorated and he kept coming up with excuses not to do it.

"Did you know about all of this as well?" I asked John astonished.

It transpired that all of my family had planned and paid for this wonderful surprise and everyone knew about it, even my neighbours. It seemed the only person that didn't know was me.

On entering Professor Cooke's clinic for one of my frequent checkups, John and I took a seat whilst we waited for my name to be called. Jean had been there that day and we happily chatted as I waited for the Professor Cooke to attend to me.

Professor Cooke was truly an amazing individual that I had come to know well and admired so much. I recalled how Alison had once told me that he was a keen extreme skier, something that had brought an instant smile to my face, given that he most definitely was the wrong side of fifty. I was never that sure if Alison had only been pulling my leg when she told me this, not that I would ever find out because I don't think I would have ever plucked up the courage to come right out and ask him. So instead I would just recall my surgeon's words periodically and have a little giggle to myself at the vision of Professor Cooke in a ski suit racing down a mountain.

My name was now being called; I got to my feet and began to make my way to one of the many treatment rooms. No one had to explain to me what would happen next, given that the clinic was now an all too familiar part of my life. Going over to the bed that was situated in the middle of the room, I automatically pulled the screens that surrounded it and in no time at all had stripped to the waist and donned the hospital gown that had been left for me.

Shortly after, the screens were pulled slightly back and in walked Professor Cooke.

"How have you been keeping?" he asked me.

"Getting there," I told him.

That seemed to be my answer to everyone these days when asked how I was feeling. After examining me fully and telling me that everything appeared to be fine, he stood momentarily in front of me before then going on to say,

"No, how are you really feeling Roseann?"

"Well Prof," I said, "there are people out there that are walking about like little time bombs that have cancer and are totally unaware of that fact. Then there are those who leave their house at the beginning of a day never to return to their loved ones because they have been tragically killed. Others sadly have to face the fact that nothing else can be done to save them, as well as the fact that their death is so frightfully imminent. I, on the other hand, am one of the lucky ones. I know that everything is being done that can possibly be done to help me. You and almost everyone else involved in my care have all given me 110%. What more can I ask for?"

At that, Professor Cooke looked directly into my eyes and smiled; no other words were needed. I felt good that day at being able to openly share my feelings in a special way with such a remarkable man. Just the word "Thanks" can mean so much to someone or bring brightness to a darkened day.

"Hooray!" I thought to myself as I sat in the clinic waiting to receive my last chemotherapy treatment. I had successfully got through the past 9 months and lived to tell the tale, something that at times a felt I would never do.

Looking back, it was hard to believe that for three quarters of a year my body had been constantly bombarded by chemotherapy. Reflecting over that time, I found myself amazed at how my body had managed to cope with the beatings it had endured. I was so very, very pleased with myself and even Veronica could not take that feeling away from me.

"Only a few more appointments," I told myself and then I could close this chapter of my life knowing that I had conquered it successfully. Two major hurdles in my fight to survive; a truly emotional experience.

As John and I left the clinic that day I told him, "A day for celebration I think." After all I did have something to celebrate wouldn't you say?

Chapter Nineteen

It Was a Privilege to Call Her My Friend

She was a wonderful person and it was an honour and a privilege to have known her. Her name was Evelyn; we first met one day at the chemotherapy clinic. I do not know what attracted us to each other, but on that day we just seem to sail into conversation. She, like I, had been diagnosed with breast cancer, although her diagnosis had been made approximately 12 years previously. The reason for her attending the oncology clinic was because her cancer had now spread to her lungs, liver and bones.

When we were talking one day, I had told her of a poem that my sister, an exceptional writer of verse, had written for me about a cancer bunny that ate cancer carrots. Evelyn seemed intrigued by what I had told her, so much so that I had promised to bring her a copy of my poem the next time I returned to the clinic.

"If you are not here, I will leave it in an envelope with your name on it at the reception desk," I told her.

As it happened, it would be another month before I would see Evelyn again. On walking into the clinic, I instantly noticed her sitting talking to her friend Anne who would on occasions come to the clinic with her. As I caught her eye she asked me, "Have you got your cancer bunny yet?" Puzzled, I waited for her to explain further. "Your cancer bunny; have you got it yet? I've got mine. He sits at the side of my bed along with the copy of the poem you gave me," she continued.

Cancer No Not Me!

"No," I told her. To be honest the penny still hadn't dropped as to what she was trying to tell me.

However, things began to become clearer as she then went on to explain in further detail what she was talking about. It transpired that she had got a toy furry bunny and this was her own special bunny that ate her cancer carrots.

"What a fantastic idea," I told her.

She told me how my sister's poem had been such a tremendous help to her.

"I'll get you one," she promised. "The next time I come to the clinic, I will bring you your very own cancer bunny," she said.

True to her word, the next time I went to the clinic there he was; my very own cancer bunny. He was white with a purple polka dot jacket and purple check pantaloons, with very long legs and a lovely pale blue ribbon tied in a bow around his neck. He certainly brought a smile to my face when I saw him for the first time.

"Oscar; that's what I will call him," I told myself.

When I returned home that day, the first thing I did was to take my cancer bunny and place him at the side of my bed, just as Evelyn had with her bunny.

Often, when I was feeling exhausted or rather low, I would go and lie on the top of my bed and in my imagination I would visualise Oscar busily running around inside my body eating all, if any, cancer carrots that he would find. It was truly a great way to generate positive thinking and it would give me a great sense of comfort knowing that I could mentally obliterate any little cancer seeds that might be lurking in my body.

When I next saw Evelyn, I told her how I would go through my little ritual of sending Oscar in search of cancer carrots. We both laughed at how our bunny rabbits had now became so very important to us.

Cancer No Not Me!

Let me share my sister's poem with you.

Thought Power

There's a little cancer bunny
Hiding deep inside of you
And he's hunting cancer carrots;
They're his favourite things to chew.

When you lay down to rest,
That's his favourite time to play;
Just imagine him so happy
As he chews cancer away.

He's getting even stronger
As you help him track them down.
Can't you see him growing bigger,
Every time he is around?

So whenever you are lonely
Or you just have a bad day,
Release the cancer bunny
And let him out to play.

I know it's just a mind game
But with faith it really works,
So fill up the cancer bunny ... .
Imagination never hurts.

As Evelyn and I became closer, our friendship blossomed and we would share our time together telling each other all about our lives. Evelyn had told me how she had set up a charity and had raised a substantial amount of money for breast cancer.

"I've met a few famous people and have even walked down a catwalk with Naomi Campbell," she said proudly.

I was amazed by the energy that seemed to naturally flow from her and listened intently to her stories of all the things she had achieved since being diagnosed with breast cancer.

"I've started to write a book about my life since being diagnosed with cancer," she told me one day. "I haven't got very far, but if you want to read it I would be happy to bring it in for you."

I really felt rather proud at being given the opportunity to read such a personal piece of literature and told her if she did not mind, I would love to read her work.

I could not wait to get home the day that she handed it to me so that I could read it. I was almost like a child that had been given a precious gift as I sat on the sofa at home and slowly opened the envelope that Evelyn had given me. Her book told of how she had been married with two children, a boy and a girl. It hadn't been a happy marriage and by the sound of it her husband was a bit of a waste of space and had given Evelyn a hard time.

On being diagnosed with her breast cancer, she had decided that she was not going to live an unhappy life any longer. Taking her two children, she sought refuge in a homeless unit, leaving her husband behind. I remember thinking as I read those words of how remarkable Evelyn really was. To be told she had cancer and on top of that choosing to change her life so dramatically, must certainly take a hell of a lot of guts.

The story of her life went on to tell of how she would often go across to the bar opposite from the homeless unit to use the telephone as there wasn't one in her accommodation. On a few occasions, she had noticed a man at the bar who would smile at her. Given that she was never one for going into pubs, let alone talking to strangers, she would smile shyly back at this person, then leave without saying a word.

As time went on, however, gradually they began to get to know each other. Initially it was with this chap asking her to join him for a drink. This lead on to them sharing an evening at his house over a meal and from then their relationship blossomed and eventually they set up home together. I felt moved as I read her short but amazing story. They were still very much a happy couple when I met Evelyn and her love for this man was truly apparent when she spoke of him.

Evelyn fought hard against her cancer but the constant toil that the chemotherapy treatments were taking on her body gradually got too much for her. She decided enough was enough and chose to stop any further treatment. She died in a homeopathic hospital, her room overlooking tranquil grounds, in the presence of her loving family. She knew when it was time for her to die and told her family she was ready. Peacefully she slipped away.

Lorne her sister telephoned me to tell me of Evelyn's passing.

"I will understand if you do not attend the funeral. I know how hard it would be for you to attend. I have watched Evelyn so many times lose friends to cancer and have seen the heartache and despair she went through at their passing."

I telephoned my mother after speaking to Evelyn's sister and on hearing my mother's voice, I just broke down and cried as I told her of Evelyn's death.

I decided that I would not attend Evelyn's funeral. I don't think I could have coped. Instead, I sat in my own house and at the time of her funeral service I lit a candle for her, something that I still do to this day every dawn of a new year. Evelyn was truly my inspiration.

Chapter Twenty

Time for a Radiotherapy Suntan

The day of my first radiotherapy treatment had arrived. I was to see a Dr MacMillan at clinic four in the Glasgow Royal Infirmary. Given that this was also around the time when I was due to attend the chemotherapy clinic to have my bloods checked for the very last time, I had arranged both appointments for the same afternoon. I had now became a master at shuffling my appointments and felt rather pleased at having got my timings down to a fine art.

Arriving at clinic four with John by my side, I automatically headed for the reception desk to inform them that I had arrived. Handing over the letter that had been sent to me instructing me to attend, I then waited whilst the receptionist double checked my details.

"That's fine Mrs Gallagher. If you would like to take a seat in the waiting area until your name is called," she said.

Sitting next to John, I found myself scanning the faces of the other people in the clinic as I wondered if they were also there for the same reason as I was. Surprisingly, none had the usual telltale signs of having been through chemotherapy. I thought that maybe they had had a type of chemotherapy treatment that didn't cause their hair to fall out. I tried to make sense of the fact that I appeared to be the only person with a bandana to mask my hair loss.

An hour passed and John and I sifted through the usual hospital magazines, as in the background people's names were called. Then we would watch as each person disappeared into the treatment area, only to lift our heads not long after, to watch them after having apparently been seen by the doctor. Both of us found it rather strange that my name had still not been mentioned, but knew from experience that you could have a lengthy wait in clinics such as these.

Another hour went by and still we waited. By this time it was nearly 4pm. Enough was enough. I caught the attention of a nurse who was obviously working in the clinic. Enquiring if she had any idea how long it would be before I would be seen, she asked, "What is your name?" On telling her, she seemed none the wiser as to whom I was.

"I gave my details to your receptionist when I arrived," I told her.

She went over to the girl at the reception desk, only to return rather sheepishly as she apologetically informed me that the receptionist had not put my name forward. To say I was incensed was an understatement, but what could I do?

"I will ensure that you are seen shortly," the nurse stressed.

True to her word, not long after the nurse returned and called out my name.

As both John and I entered the consultation room, we were met by a rather small man of around 50 who instantly introduced himself as Doctor MacMillan. Without taking the time to offer us a seat, he began to inform me how he would be unable to discuss my treatment. I couldn't believe it. John and I had waited hours to see this man and now he was telling me it had all been for nothing. Continuing, he informed me that he did not have my case notes, so how was he expected to do his job if the information he needed was not available?

Both John and I stood there not quite knowing what to do.

"The only way I can discuss your case is if I have your case notes. I have told my nurse to contact your chemotherapy clinic and we have now found out that your records are there," he ranted, before he went on to tell us that if I wanted my consultation to go ahead that day then we would have to collect my case notes from the clinic and bring them back to him.

John's lips were white with anger and I could tell that he was only moments away from erupting. If it wasn't for the fact that I was practically embedding my fingernails into his hand as a way of pleading with him not to say anything, God only knows what would have happened.

By the time I reached the chemotherapy clinic, my emotions were all over the place and once seated I could feel tears begin to fill my eyes. I was so upset at what had happened and how this man had managed to make me feel as if I were nothing more other than a bit of dirt on his shoe. By the time Veronica handed me my case notes, I had lost it.

"There is no way I will accept being spoken to like that. I think that some professionals in this hospital forget that it is people like me that keep them in a job. How dare he!" I bemoaned.

Veronica tried her best to calm me down. I think I had shocked her in the way that I had reacted, given that I had never openly complained. If anything, I made a point of praising most of the people involved in my care. By this time, Veronica had taken us into the doctor's room in the clinic.

"I am going to report him," I told her.

I will give Veronica her due that day; she tried her best to resolve the situation.

"Please talk to Doctor MacMillan, Roseann, and tell him how much he has upset you. Really that is the best way to deal with this situation. The last thing you need is to go home tonight angered by something that can so easily be dealt with," she said.

"We'll see," I told her.

Making our way back to clinic four, I thought long and hard about what Veronica had said and I had to admit that for once she was right. Why should I go home feeling miserable when I could deal with the problem there and then? By the time we had returned to the clinic, the receptionist had packed up and the place was almost empty. On seeing that we had returned, the nurse that I had spoken to earlier once again showed us into the consultation room.

My heart was pounding and I felt sick at the thought of the confrontation that was about to take place, but I had made up my mind there was no going back; I was going to let this man know just how much he had upset me.

Sitting at his desk, Doctor MacMillan spoke first.

"Well, Mrs Gallagher, I can now discuss your treatment with you," to which I replied in a rather abrupt way, "No, Dr MacMillan. I know that there are a lot of people like me in the world and there are very few people like you," I told him. "I can appreciate that you have a lot of people to see and so little time in which to see them. However, that does not give you the right to speak to me in the manner you did and as I have told Veronica my chemotherapy nurse, I am intending to put a letter of complaint into the hospital about your manner and the way in which you have treated me. It was not my fault that you did not have my case notes; it is your responsibility to ensure that you have the appropriate paperwork at hand for your clinic, not mine."

There, I had said it and in a polite, but assertive manner. I was now no longer upset, nor did I feel intimidated. I had successfully dealt with the matter and it was now he who felt rather uncomfortable

Apologising for the way in which he had spoken to me, Doctor MacMillan went on to say that it had not been his intention to upset me.

"I am only one man, working alone in a very busy clinic," he said.

Telling him I could appreciate that he had a difficult job, I pointed out that if he had taken the time to explain that he had not been able to obtain my notes and then informed me that he would send someone to collect them, I would have happily waited whilst he got things in order.

In the end, he briefly when over what my treatment entailed, then informed me that he would contact me by post with a date for me to attend the radiotherapy department at the Beatson hospital. He then shook both my hand and John's before again apologising for any misunderstanding. I felt so much better on leaving the hospital that day, knowing that I had found the strength to challenge someone with regard to their actions.

With my encounter with Doctor MacMillan firmly put to the back of my mind, I tried now only to focus on my next hurdle; that of the removal of my Hickman line. I felt extremely apprehensive, especially after being told by one of the chemotherapy doctors that this procedure would be done without an anaesthetic and at the clinic. Knowing that there was nothing I could do to change that fact, I tried now only to think of good thoughts and of how wonderful it would be to no longer have two plastic tubes protruding from my body. Then again, without my Hickman line I would no longer require the services of my wonderful district nurse and that was a little daunting, since she had played such a major role in seeing me through many of the difficult times that I had experienced in the past. I felt as though one of my imaginary safety nets was about to be taken from beneath me.

I felt terrified as I walked through the doors of the clinic that day and even more uncomfortable at the thought of having to endure my experience in such an open and impersonal environment. I recalled my past thoughts about how unfair the lack of privacy must have seemed to individuals who had to tolerate having their very personal details and treatments being shared with everyone in the clinic. I was now the person who felt uncomfortable at knowing that every word spoken during the removal of my Hickman line would be openly shared. My nerves increased even more as I worried about not being able to remain composed, or embarrassing myself by openly crying.

The receptionist informed me that they were ready to see me. Being met by Doctor Grey, I must admit, made me feel slightly less nervous, given that I had seen her on numerous occasions and we got on well.

"You'll be glad to get shot of this," she joked as she prepared a trolley with the things that she would require to remove my line.

I didn't reply, but managed a rather unsure smile. Seeing how nervous I appeared, Doctor Grey reassuringly told me that the whole procedure would only take a few minutes and that before I knew it I would be on my way home.

"Thank God," I told myself.

After manoeuvring myself into an upright sitting position on the bed as instructed, I then waited for the doctor to begin. I couldn't believe that within a matter of seconds the two stitches that held my Hickman line in place had been cut and I was now being told by Doctor Grey to take a very deep breath.

"Now all you have to do is breathe out as I remove the line," she continued.

With that, she placed a palm on my chest just below the site of my line, then firmly leaning against my body removed my tubes in one quick motion. Maintaining the pressure with her palm on my chest, Doctor Grey then informed me that apart from having to lean on my chest for a few more minutes, all that remained was for me to relax for the next half hour with no sudden movements. Then, if all appeared well, I could go on my merry way. All that worry for nothing and into the bargain I hadn't made a fool of myself by shouting out or crying, much to my relief.

Over the next few days, major changes occurred in my life. No longer did I have to go through the procedure of a line flush every second day. I also no longer required many of the drugs that had been a big part of my daily life, because my bloods were once again on the up. To make matters even better, the problems that I had experienced in getting my pain under control had now also been made so much easier to tolerate, due to a change in medication. To top that, Isabell had informed me that she would still be popping in to see how I was doing on a regular basis.

I'm not saying that everything in the garden was totally rosy, but it was a hell of a lot brighter. Very gradually, the "sick" me was gradually being peeled away to reveal the person I once was, not as before, but even better. Even my hair was slowly beginning to re-grow, which was really uplifting.

Halloween had arrived and so had all the excitement associated with "trick or treat". The reason for my enthusiasm at the arrival of this day was due to the fact that I had decided that my granddaughters and I would dress up and go in search of goodies at our neighbours' doors.

"Too right; life is for living and I am going to share as many magical moments as I can with the girls," I told John, who was looking at me as though I were mad.

The girls were all for it when I had told them that I was also going to dress up.

"What will you be Gran?" they both asked, almost in unison.

On telling them that I had decided to be a pumpkin, they both looked at each other then giggled excitedly. Little did I know just how much my actions had meant to my youngest granddaughter until she telephoned me a few days later to inform me that she was going to be a pumpkin just like her gran.

"Well, you can be a baby pumpkin and I will be the mummy pumpkin," I told her, her actions almost bringing a tear to my eye.

It felt good to have this new air of confidence and a carefree manner that now enabled me to do things that I would have never dreamed of doing in the past, either because I would be far too worried about what people would think, or because I might embarrass myself. But none of that mattered now; it was what I wanted that was now important and that was sharing priceless moments with my granddaughters as they grew up.

Telling my sister Debbie of my intention, I was surprised to find that I had also rekindled the child in her as she excitedly told me that she too would bring her children along and would also like to dress up and go trick or treating.

"I'll be a clown," she told me, ecstatic at the thought.

My house was a full of laughter that night as all six of us donned our outfits in preparation for our night of fun.

Even John had to admit that my idea was nothing less than wonderful when he saw just how excited the children were. I must admit we all looked rather spectacular; a mummy and baby pumpkin, a beautiful princess, a genie with a magic lamp, a clown and the Grim Reaper, no less.

I tell you, the faces of the children ringing our doorbell to trick or treat, was priceless. They just stood there open mouthed until we cajoled them from their hypnotic state by asking them whether they were going to sing or tell a joke in order to receive their goody bag. I'm sure we had double the amount of kids at our door than the doors of our neighbours, as word quickly got around that two women had dressed up and were actually going to go out for their Halloween.

Walking down the street attracted many a stare, but heads held high, we carried on regardless. Going from one door to another seemed to attract kids from all nooks and crannies and before I knew it I appeared to have my own tribe of little people. There must have been at least twenty kids following in my footsteps and when we knocked on a door, the person answering it was literally bowled over by the vastness of our group. What a night and I loved every minute of it!

The first day of my attendance at the Radiotherapy Unit at the Beatson Oncology had arrived. In a letter that I had received a few days earlier, I was instructed that on arrival I should report to the simulator department. I didn't have clue what exactly that meant and my apprehension spilled over as I nervously bombarded John with questions that I knew he would be unable to answer.

"Do you think that means that I will receive my first treatment? How long do you think I will be there?"

Cancer No Not Me!

To tell you the truth, I think I just needed to hear John tell me that I had nothing to worry about and that everything would be fine.

"Do you want me to come with you?" John asked, knowing that my mother had almost insisted that she would be my escort for that day.

How I wanted to say "Yes", but I knew I couldn't. My mother had looked upon this day with pride at knowing that she would be right there by my side to look after me. I couldn't take that important role away from her and that's just what I would be doing if I had asked John to come with us.

"No, mum will look after me," I lied.

On arriving at the hospital, I made my way to the main reception area at the entrance of the building and on handing over the letter that I had received, I then waited to be told what to do next. Mother put her arm in mine, almost as if she was trying her best to ease any feeling of nervousness that I might have been experiencing.

"I'm alright Mum," I reassured her. "Let's face it; surely it can't be any worse than the chemotherapy treatments," I continued.

We stood in silence as my details were fed into a computer. After handing me back the letter containing my details, the receptionist then proceeded to give me directions on how to get to the department I was to attend. My mother and I walked off arm in arm in search of it.

As we walked through the entrance of the simulator department, I was overwhelmed by the massive waiting area, but even more taken aback by the amount of people that were seated in it. On handing my details over to yet another receptionist, I was then instructed to take a seat and told that my name would be called when they were ready for me.

Instantly, I began to look for any signs that would lead me to the actual role of this department, but I remained oblivious. Slowly casting my eyes over all the people in the room, I was intrigued to find just how wide the age differences of my fellow patients were. There appeared to be some who looked as young as twenty and then others who were very much older; in their eighties maybe. What amazed me more though, was how they all sat there in silence as they waited for their names to be called.

As my name was called, I automatically got up from the chair and made my way towards the nurse who was scanning the room in search of me.

"I won't be too long," I told my mother, as I gave her hand a quick squeeze.

Strangely enough, I can't really say that I felt scared at that moment, just a little more apprehensive at not knowing what to expect. With a large smile, the nurse introduced herself and then asked that I follow as she directed me to a door at the far left of the waiting area. With one last quick look round to make sure my mother was alright, I entered the room.

No wonder there was no information to tell you what exactly an appointment to the simulator room entailed, as I found it hard to believe my eyes. Right in the centre of this room was a machine that looked as if it had just come out of a science fiction movie; it was huge. By this time my thought processes were running at an alarming rate, as were the butterflies that fluttered wildly around my stomach. Trying to take in everything that surrounded me, I could see that part of the room was sectioned off by a door with a long glass partition, which had approximately four people behind it.

There was an operating theatre type table also in the centre of the room directly underneath this monster of a machine. My nerves were obviously apparent to the nurse.

"Don't worry Mrs Gallagher; what you are having done today is totally painless. I know it all looks rather frightening, but honestly you won't be long in here."

"Thank God for that," I thought.

"What exactly am I having done today?" I asked her.

"Oh, I am sorry Mrs Gallagher for not explaining to you. I had automatically assumed that you had been told and were fully aware of what will happen," she apologised.

My mind went back to my consultation with Doctor MacMillan, but I could not recall being told about this. I knew this was certainly something that I would have remembered.

The nurse explained that what I was looking at was a simulator machine and that its job was to basically map out exactly were on my body my radiotherapy treatments should be administered. This was done by feeding all the data relating to me and my planned treatments into the machine. After receiving the information, it would then plan a structured set of coordinates for the radiographer responsible for administering my treatments.

"With this new information we then mark your body with a few small tattoos to ensure that your treatment remains accurate and precise. Therefore, on every day that you attend for your radiotherapy treatment, all this information will be fed into the radiotherapy machine to locate the exact coordinates, as well as how long and where each treatment should be given," she said.

Although that was a lot to take in, I was certainly much more relaxed once this had been explained to me. As I gave an almighty sigh of relief, the nurse laughed then said,

Cancer No Not Me!

"Told you it wasn't that bad."

Lying on the table stripped to the waist as instructed, I waited for the mapping of my body to begin. No longer did I feel any anxiety. I only wish I could say the same for my poor mother who I knew would be worrying sick about me.

After the nurse had been joined by two of her colleagues, all three then began the process of moving my body into the required position. A foam cushion was placed under my left shoulder and then a metal bar was positioned directly behind my head. Once everything was in place, I was then asked to lift my left arm up and over my head and grasp a metal bar, which had been clamped to the table directly behind my head. It was all rather technical really, although I must say that I believed the process was made a whole lot easier by the fact that I let the nurses position me exactly how they wanted, rather than trying to do it myself.

Shortly after, Dr MacMillan entered the room, which strangely enough took me by surprise because he was the last person I expected to see that day. After acknowledging my presence, he then turned his attention to the nurses and began giving what seemed like instructions. To tell you the truth, he could have been speaking in a foreign language for all I knew because I didn't understand one word that came from his lips. Standing with his arms folded, he then watched whilst further changes were made to my position. After appearing satisfied that the apparent modifications had been made, Dr MacMillan and the nurses then left through the adjoining door, only to appear moments later behind the glass partition.

Lying there alone, I looked at this massive machine that was now suspended only inches away from my body. I began to wonder how in the world someone could actually invent, design and put together such an intricate piece of equipment. Without warning, the machine took on a life of its own and began to manoeuvre itself in a robotic fashion in many different directions, as it apparently ran through the different stages of its programme. Just as unexpectedly as it had started, it came to a complete stop.

Joined once again by Dr MacMillan and the nurses, I then lay waiting to be told what would happen next; not that there was much more left to do. A few moments later I was quickly marked with three small tattoos on the area of my body that would be treated with radiotherapy. I was informed that my experience in the simulator department was now over, as two of the nurses then began to help me get up from the table.

On leaving the room, one of the nurses stopped me in my tracks.

"The doctor has still to meet with you to go over some things relating to your treatment. If you would like to take a seat in the waiting area, he will be with you shortly," she told me.

The last thing I wanted was a one to one chat with Dr MacMillan. I was certain that he would bring up our exchange of words and began to feel nervous once more. Now I was truly wishing that I had brought John along.

Joining my mother in the waiting area, I told her what had happened during my time in the simulator room.

"All that is left for me to do is have a quick meeting with the doctor to discuss my treatment, then we can go home," I explained.

Not once did I reveal to my mother how increasingly nervous I was now becoming, given the fact that I would be unable to take my mother into the meeting with me for moral support. I hadn't told her of the previous encounter with this doctor, because I had not wanted to worry her.

On calling my name, Dr MacMillan then escorted me to one of the vacant consultation rooms. After asking me to take a seat, he then sat down himself.

"Firstly Mrs Gallagher, let me again apologise for the misunderstanding between us on our first meeting," he said.

"There is no further need to apologise; the matter is now closed," I told him, as I tried hard to mask the fact that I felt uncomfortable at having to see him on my own.

Thankfully, the conversation had now turned to the topic of my radiotherapy treatment. It was explained to me that I would be required to sign a consent form, not unlike the one that has to be completed by a patient before going for any type of surgical procedure. Continuing, Doctor MacMillan then informed me that as I had decided against having reconstruction surgery, this meant that I would be able to receive my radiotherapy over twenty treatments instead of thirty. Apparently, it had something to do with the intensity of the treatment affecting the texture and suppleness of the skin. Therefore, those who had opted for reconstruction would receive their radiotherapy treatment over a period of thirty treatments to reduce the damage to the skin's elasticity.

By now, I was feeling quite relaxed and pleased in the knowledge that this next stage of treatment had been cut by a third, although little did I know this would only be short lived as Dr MacMillan then went on to inform me that three areas of my body would require treatment. "Your chest wall, neck and underarm," he told me.

His words instantly made me feel uneasy. I had never for one minute envisaged that I would need treatment in more than one place. Not much else registered after that; all I could think about was the fact that I now believed that instead of taking one step forward, I was in actual fact taking two steps back. Those oh so familiar feelings of doubt had re-emerged.

"That's it, we are all finished," I told my mum as I tried to force a smile.

I didn't feel much like smiling. All I wanted to do was get home as quickly as possible, knowing that I so desperately needed to share my fears with John before these morbid thoughts had a chance to overwhelm me again. I knew he would reassure me that everything would be alright.

How right I was about John that day. After only being in his presence for a short period of time, he had successfully helped me to accept my situation as it stood and showed me the benefits of the treatments that had first caused me to become concerned.

"They obviously think that by covering every conceivable angle, they are not only holding your best interests at heart, but I assume they also hope to reduce your chances of reoccurrence. There is no way they would even consider this course of action if they had not felt that its outcome would be favourable. If I were you, I would be feeling relieved at knowing I was getting more as opposed to less," he said reassuringly.

He certainly did having the knack of turning a negative thought into a positive one. Looking at it from that perspective, I could now see the logic behind the decision. I don't know where I would have been without John. He truly instilled faith in me at times when I felt a situation was at its worst, or I was at my lowest.

A fortnight later, I was walking through the doors of the Beatson Oncology Centre for my first course of radiotherapy treatment. After going through the usual process of informing the main reception desk of my arrival, I played the waiting game once more. I felt great relief in knowing that John was by my side to take in all the information of how to get to the radiotherapy department, because by then my nerves were heightening and I was becoming increasingly anxious about what lay ahead.

Before I knew it, we were on the move again. All I could do was hold tightly onto John's hand as he directed me through a series of corridors. It's strange, but instinct told me we had reached our destination as I lifted my head to glance at the writing above the doorway we were on the verge of stepping through. The waiting area was rather small and square, but it appeared to link to a long corridor that had all manner of electrical and computer equipment running along the right side of it. About three doors along on the left, there was something that could not have been missed; copious amounts of hazard warning signs. On noticing a woman who looked as if she was a member of staff, I approached her and practically thrust my letter of introduction into her hand. Nerves had now seriously taken control over my body and it was as if I was on autopilot, going through a series of motions subconsciously.

"Take a seat and someone will be with you shortly," the woman said.

As John and I sat down, I looked around at the other people waiting. There was a woman of around sixty-five in her dressing gown who had been wheeled in on a trolley just after us and was most probably from one of the wards within the building. Then there was a young couple who were sitting near the doorway. You didn't have to guess who had come there that day for treatment; you just had to look at the young man and his lack of hair and scarring on his head to know the answer to that question. Looking at this poor boy, who appeared to be in his very early twenties, I began to realise how lucky I was in that I had at least got to 39 years of age. Two other women of around fifty sat chatting rather loudly about their treatments and how many they each had left to go. I listened hard to their conversation, almost praying that one of them would mention exactly what radiotherapy treatment entailed, but no such luck.

I watched as one of the nurses approached from the far end of the adjoining corridor.

"Roseann Gallagher," she called out once she had reached the waiting area.

I felt childlike and scared as I got to my feet and quietly confirmed, "That's me."

On directing me to a rail that held a large row of terry towelling dressing gowns, she explained that every person that attended for the duration of their treatment were all given their own individual gown, identifiable by a large white tag pinned to the collar.

"If you would like to have a look, there should be one there for you," she said.

Going through the row of gowns, it didn't take me long to locate the one with my name clearly marked in bold black writing. The nurse then asked me to follow her.

"Bring the dressing gown with you," she said, as she lead me to the top end of the corridor.

After being shown to a patients' changing room, she instructed me to strip to the waist and don my gown. Sitting on one of two chairs at the far end of the corridor, I felt rather lost as I waited to meet the person who would be responsible for coordinating my treatment. Quickly, my eyes looked down the corridor in the hope of seeing John. I was overwhelmed with love for him when I saw that he had actually changed his seat and was now positioned directly facing up the corridor and was waving his hand to let me know he was as near to me as was allowed. It's amazing how little things mean such a lot. John's actions seemed to spark an inner confidence within me, giving me the strength to believe, as he did, in my ability to take in my stride whatever lay ahead that day.

Taking in my surroundings, I noticed that there was a small passageway that extended beyond the corridor; its entrance was clearly marked with, a "No entry" sign and red warnings signs covering the walls, ceiling and floor. There was also what appeared to be a work station or inlay filled with an array of electrical equipment and computer software. There was a monitor with a screen that was divided into four individual pictures, all of which focused on a metal table from different angles. They obviously monitored the person having radiotherapy via close circuit television. Stacked high on the work surface where all this apparatus sat was a rather large pile of patients' medical case notes.

My name being spoken brought me back to reality, as I turned to see a woman of around forty appear from the entrance of the passageway that donned all the danger signs.

"Mrs Gallagher, would you like to come through?" she said.

Giving a half hearted smile, I got to my feet and followed as requested. Entering a vast room at the end of the passageway, I found it very similar to that of the simulator room I had visited a few weeks earlier, although I would say that there may have been a bit more machinery in this one. On being asked to remove my gown, I was then instructed to lie down on a metal table in the centre of the room. It's hard

Cancer No Not Me!

to explain, but the minute I removed this gown exposing the upper half of my body, a feeling of vulnerability overpowered me and I found myself instinctively wrapping my arms around my chest in a frantic effort to hide the parts of my body now so openly exposed.

As I began to walk towards the table, another female member of staff entered the room, which made me feel even more exposed. Without acknowledging my presence, she quickly began to position and clamp a metal pole at the head of the table, then stood with foam pads in her hand in preparation to position them under my left shoulder once I had placed myself on the table. It was like a mirror image of what had been done during my time in the simulator room. After assisting me to position myself, a square jelly like pad was placed over the area of my body that was to be treated with radiotherapy.

"Now don't move, we need you to stay in that position," one of the radiographers emphasised.

Without another word, both of the women left the room. Once again, I found myself alone with a huge machine not unlike the simulator suspended only inches away from my body. I felt terrified. I did try my best to relax, but that was almost impossible as I found myself alone and with no knowledge of what was about to happen to me.

"Now your treatment is about to begin. Do not move," a disembodied voice informed me via a speaker that hung on one of the walls.

Shortly after, the machine begun to rotate, then changed direction and made a sound similar to that of a digital camera continuously clicking. I tried my best to focus only on the fact that it was imperative that I remained still.

"Please hurry up," I found myself silently pleading, as my arm and neck ached due to the position I was in.

Cancer No Not Me!

It was such a relief when the machine came to a complete stop and I was once again joined by both radiographers.

"Can I move now?" I asked, the instant they entered the room.

One of the women told me that I could, but only for a few moments as I would be required to go through the whole procedure again, not once more but twice, before my course of treatment for the day had been completed. So once again the machine was re-programmed for my next treatment and the whole process started and finished in a similar fashion.

With only one more treatment to go, I gave a quick sigh of relief, before the machine once again began to spin and turn and end up within inches from my body. Suddenly, I began to panic, as without warning the thin jelled square that had been placed over the site to be treated with radiotherapy began to slowly slip down the side of my body. I began to panic and wondered what I should do. "Do I move? No, mustn't move. God, will the machine burn me if this pad falls from my body?" I felt well and truly trapped as my panic increased.

Looking around the room as my heart raced, I caught sight of a monitor with numbers clearly visible; 55 then 54 – it seemed to be reducing a second at a time. Quickly, I realised that this was the time that remained of my treatment. I had this terrible urge of wanting to instinctively jump off of the table as all the while this pad just kept slowly moving down my body. I silently pleaded for the treatment to finish before I ended up with no protection from the rays of this machine. The jelly square was by now halfway down my chest wall and felt that at any moment it would fall to the floor. All the while I could hear in my head the words of the radiographer, "Don't move; you have to remain completely still". I was almost frantic by the time the machine eventually stopped.

When both women again appeared in the room, I almost cried as I told them how the pad had begun to move slowly down my body and how I had been terrified that at any moment I would be severely burned.

"I didn't know whether I should get off the table or stay still as instructed," I told them, panic clearly noticeable in my voice.

"No, you don't move if that happens. In fact, it doesn't really matter whether or not the pad is placed over the area of your body being treated by radiotherapy," one of the women informed me.

I only wish she had taken the time to tell me this beforehand; it would certainly have saved me the terrible distress that I experienced over one square sheet of jelly.

If I had also been told beforehand that when the radiographers exited the room the door's warning bells would sound and also that the machine would make a noise, it would certainly have helped to ease my fears.

Complacency and possibly confidence I believe can sometimes contribute to some individuals going through the motions of their designated job like automatons. It seems the more familiar some individuals become in relation to their job, the more they just go through the motions without even giving the patient a second thought. Some tend to forget at times that what they regard as par for the course, is not the case in the eyes of a patient. Both radiographers were competent and efficient in every way, but neither took the time to offer reassurance or explain little things that they themselves felt were either obvious, or a triviality. From a patient's perspective, however, the experience of a radiotherapy unit is both alien and really rather scary. So, if you happen to be one of those who work with people, please ensure that from this day forth you now take time to spare a thought for those of us who don't understand. It only takes a few minutes, but those few minutes make the difference between someone experiencing fear at the unknown, or obtaining an understanding of those things out of the norm. In the eyes of the patient, your actions may instil feelings of confidence and respect in you and the work that you do. The person who requires radiotherapy treatment is literally putting their life in your hands, so knowing that the person responsible for your treatment empathises with your situation, means so much.

The relief I felt once I had arrived home was tremendous; such a weight had been lifted from my shoulders. No longer would I now beat myself up emotionally over the unknown area of radiotherapy; I had overcome that hurdle. My twenty radiotherapy treatments would be given from Monday to Friday for four weeks. It was also explained to me that in some cases people can experience breaks in the skin and blistering. I crossed my fingers and hoped that I would not be one of those people. I was reassured that if I developed any skin problems due to my treatment, there were clinical nurses that specialised in this area that I would see on a weekly basis, or at my request, should I be concerned or experience any problems that I felt needed addressing immediately.

My mum was on the telephone not long after my return from hospital that day to make sure that I was alright and that everything had gone according to plan. She had worried herself sick at not knowing what would actually be done to me that day.

"Remember, if you need me to go with you daughter, just pick up the phone," she told me.

Cancer No Not Me!

It's really strange; although I dearly wanted to actively involve my mother, something inside of me wanted to keep her at a distance. Maybe that protective mode we can all go into with regard to the ones we love had something to do with it. But really, when I think about it in greater depth, every time my mother accompanied me to my hospital and clinic appointments, she would always appear anxious and sad. I could not continually put her through this emotional turmoil. Even if she did stress that she wanted to be by my side, it just wasn't fair.

Over the next three days everything seemed to be going well; as my treatments increased, so did my feelings of exhaustion and fatigue. The skin on the area of my body being treated also began to show signs of redness, especially after a session of radiotherapy. It was nothing that caused me to feel concerned, however, for as the day went on the redness would gradually diminish.

On a few occasions, I had even begun to acknowledge fellow patients whom I had seen on more than one occasion. We would greet each other with a "Hello" and even sometimes discuss what treatment we were receiving and for what type of cancer. Little did I know that, come Friday, my bubble would burst.

Going through the motions that by now had become a familiar part of my life, on my arrival at the radiotherapy department one day, I instinctively walked over and removed the dressing gown with my name on it, then took a seat and waited for my name to be called. My youngest sister Debbie had come with me that day. I was in good spirits, given that I would not have to attend for radiotherapy treatment over the weekend because the department was closed.

Once my name had been called and I had stripped to the waist and donned my dressing gown, I entered the radiotherapy treatment room. I then positioned myself on the table. The radiographer that I had seen every day since the start of my treatment then went through the standard procedure of preparing the different equipment that would be required. There was also another female member of staff in the room. Both talked away to each other as if I was non-existent. I did try to join in on the conversation, but with only one word replies as a way of acknowledging that I had spoken, I soon realised that neither of the women were in the least bit interested in what I had to say. I vowed that in future I would just go in and let them get on with my treatment, since I was treated as some sort of nonentity.

"You will have to raise your arm much higher than that," the regular radiographer instructed me in rather a brusque tone. On explaining that my arm would stretch no further no matter how hard I tried, this woman then began to go on in great depth about how it was imperative that I reach up and grasp the iron bar positioned at the top of my head.

"You will have to exercise and stretch that arm. Do you do any form of physiotherapy?" she asked in a condescending tone.

I refused to be spoken to in that manner, so I replied, "I actually attend a senior physiotherapist twice a week for my arm and considering that initially I could not so much as raise it in the slightest, I think that the mobility in my arm has vastly improved," I told her.

"Well you'll just have to return to the simulator room on Monday. I can't administer your treatment if you can't manoeuvre your body into the position required," she continued.

Tears began to fill my eyes as I became increasingly upset by what was happening. If I could have got away with not having to have radiotherapy, I would have been out that door like a shot.

My treatment did go ahead that day. I don't know if my position was as it should have been or not, but the radiographer went ahead anyway. I never spoke another word to either of the staff; I just kept quiet, desperate for my treatment to be completed so that I could get away. Once dressed, I was informed that I should attend the simulator room on the Monday.

"Don't come for your treatment; it will need to be re-evaluated," I was told.

Throughout the whole weekend I constantly cried over the events that had happened that Friday. My confidence had certainly taken a knock. I just couldn't get my head around the fact that this woman thought it was alright to speak to me in the way she did, not appearing in the least bit bothered at how her words or appalling lack of sensitivity had upset me. My mother on the other hand was livid.

"How dare she treat you in that way? Come Monday, I will go with you to the hospital and give her a piece of my mind," she ranted.

The rest of my family were just as angry as my mum at the way in which I had been treated. I thought John and Billy were only seconds from blowing a gasket when they heard.

"We will take you to the hospital on Monday," they both said.

But I didn't want that; I just could not face another confrontation. In the end, I reassured both John and Billy that my mother would deal with the matter, but to be honest I had no intention of pointing out this woman to my mother either. I would tell my mother that I could not see her, even if she did cross our path on Monday.

I contacted Marie that afternoon to tell her all about what had happened that morning. She too was incensed by the way that I had been treated.

"Tell her from me that if she has anything she wishes to discuss with regard to the mobility of your arm, to contact me directly," Marie advised.

I was so grateful for her support; she had helped regain some of my confidence by reiterating how hard I had worked to gain a very respectable degree of movement in my arm.

"I'm pleased at the progress you have made. Don't let this woman take away the glory of your achievement and all the hard work you've put into getting your arm mobile again," she added.

Although speaking to Marie had made me feel slightly better, I remained rather depressed that weekend and at one point had even begun to question whether or not all the upset was worth it.

On Monday morning my mother arrived at my house bright and early, guns a blazing, which was not the norm at all for my mum; she was always a very placid individual. Having said that though, when she was on a mission, there was no stopping her.

Entering the simulator room, I was met by a woman who instantly made me feel at ease. I was thankful for that following Friday's episode. Cheerily talking away to me, this woman made light conversation until the subject of my radiotherapy treatment was brought to the fore. All she did was enquire how I was managing with such an intense form of treatment, but before I knew it tears were filling my eyes and I was finding it hard to remain composed. Seeing how upset I was becoming, the woman sympathetically enquired what was wrong. That was it, before I knew it I was telling her of my experience at the radiotherapy department the previous Friday.

"After all you have been through, the last thing you needed was that. I'm so sorry for the upset you have been caused. The radiographer had no right to talk to you in that way. After all, it's no great catastrophe if you have to return to the simulator room; many people have had to come back a second time," she told me.

I felt so relieved.

Almost within a matter of minutes, the door of the simulator room swung open and the offhand radiographer entered the room. I kept quiet and didn't give her a second glance. I felt stronger now that Marie had told me to inform this woman to contact her if she felt there was a problem with my mobility, plus my conversation with the woman in the simulator room had made me realise that it was the radiographer that was in the wrong and not I.

The radiographer didn't stay long and once she had left I explained that she had been the one that had caused me to be miserable over the whole weekend. I felt so much better at having got that off my chest. Funnily enough, from that day on the radiographer changed her attitude and was always very pleasant to me when at the department for my treatment. I often wonder if the woman I had met on my second visit to the simulator room had had a word in the radiographer's ear!

Over the following week I became quite familiar with the huge radiotherapy machine, something I found rather amusing. I became acquainted with the sequence of its programme and was no longer frightened when it made a sudden movement, or hovered only inches from my body. I had also realised that by watching a certain monitor in the room I could precisely time when each treatment would end. The three areas of my body that were being treated were all exposed to radiation for different lengths of time. The difference was only a matter of a few seconds, but all the same this was something I was now aware of. At times I was rather intrigued as to why, however, I never enquired about the reasons for this, assuming it probably had something to do with where my actual cancer had been.

I was now becoming so very tired and it would not be unusual for me to go for my treatment and then spend the rest of the day and night in bed. I was also prescribed a cream known as Aqueous for the redness on my body caused by my treatment. It worked wonders and I'm sure that covering the area of my body affected twice daily with this cream definitely contributed to preventing my skin from actually breaking down or blistering. It remained very red, but really presented no other problems. I was lucky in that sense. Other patients have told me that they felt very tender and sore on and around the area of their body being treated, but with no burning sensation. Others said it was like suffering from sunburn.

Overall, I found my radiotherapy treatment painless when administered, although I must admit I was rather embarrassed when having to lie so exposed in full view on a monitor during my treatment. I often wondered if people other than the technician could also see me; maybe as they delivered a letter or cleaned the general area.

Cancer No Not Me!

Some people had to come from far and wide to receive their radiotherapy treatment and others had to be put up in a hotel Monday to Friday for the duration of their treatment because they lived too far away to commute. It must have been so hard for them to cope with having to go through their treatment alone.

On one of the days I was at the radiotherapy department, my youngest sister and I got talking to the young couple that I had noticed on my first day at the department. I had seen them on a few occasions since then, but apart from the usual polite greetings, I had never had a full conversation with them. On this day, however, the young man and I were soon in deep conversation about the types of cancer we had been diagnosed with and the surgeries and treatments we had been through. At one point all four of us were having a really good laugh about the funny things that had happened to us since being diagnosed. He enjoyed my story of the day I wore my wig and how it itched like hell.

This young man had been diagnosed with a brain tumour and had endured major brain surgery and chemotherapy. He was now receiving radiotherapy treatment. We spoke for what seemed like ages and were able to share a few tips. He told me how a friend had bought him an Aloe Vera Plant and how he would smear the sap from its leaves onto the area of his head being treated by radiotherapy.

"It's a great thing. I haven't had any bother with redness or skin breakage," he told me.

I told him of the Aqueous cream that I was using, but his plant certainly seemed a hell of a lot more effective in reducing redness and maintaining healthy skin. His head was in great condition; not a mark to be seen.

Cancer No Not Me!

I often think of that young man, hoping he successfully won his fight against cancer. He was so young and had so much to live for. Again, I reminded myself how lucky I was to have at least got to thirty-eight before being diagnosed. I never saw him or his wife after that, because our treatments never seemed to coincide.

I was now in my third week and at the halfway mark of treatments, a milestone I was glad to reach. Having to attend the hospital for my treatment on five consecutive days left me totally drained. Sometimes it took all the strength that I could muster just to get me on to my feet, let alone to the hospital, even though I had a member of my family to drive me to and fro. Telling myself that my treatment would soon be over helped, the days still dragged. Like a child counting down the days to Christmas, it just never felt that my last day of treatment would ever arrive. The fact that I still had my physiotherapy appointments with Marie twice a week was also a contributing factor to my fatigue. On few occasions I considered putting my trips to Marie on the back burner, at least until my radiotherapy treatment had been completed, but after giving it great thought I decided against it. I had come so far and achieved so much since being assigned to Marie. It was hard to believe that at one point I could only raise my arm a matter of inches, whereas now I could lift it above my head with ease and to some degree behind my back. There was no way that I was about to risk undoing all the good work we had accomplished together. She was also one of my earth angels, there when I needed her for reassurance, advice and guidance.

Isabell also remained in contact. She would pop in periodically to enquire how I coping. I was so thankful that she hadn't just cut me off once my Hickman line had been removed; another one of my earth angels, who was always there to give advice, offer reassurance and help me through the difficult times.

I still had the same person administering my radiotherapy, as well as a few other radiographers who would assist on different days. I did try on countless occasions to instigate a conversation, or attempt to join in when the staff would be busily talking whilst setting up the apparatus. Nevertheless, I always got the impression that I annoyed them when I did that, so in the end I gave up trying and just went through the motions of turning up and positioning myself on the table, only to find a few moments later that I was alone when the staff left the room without telling me. I would have truly loved to have felt at ease when I went for my radiotherapy, but I never did. It was as if the staff of that department kept themselves to themselves and only conversed with each other. Either that or maybe they just didn't particularly like me. I tried my best not to dwell on it.

If the staff had taken the time to give a thought to their patients and got to know them a bit better, I'm sure they would have derived greater job satisfaction. Well that's what I believed anyway, given my experience of working in a caring profession.

I was surprised to walk into the radiotherapy department one day and literally bump into one of the three women I had met whilst in hospital for my mastectomy; the woman who had found it extremely difficult – as did her daughters – to accept her breast cancer diagnosis.

"How are you doing?" I enquired.

On telling me that she was still cancer free, she then began to open up to me. She told me how she was finding it difficult to make ends meet.

"I applied for Disability Living Allowance but was turned down," she told me.

She looked very worried as she went on to tell me that her employer was pressurising her to either leave or return to work.

"I don't know what I'm going to do; I can't afford to lose my job. It's bad enough as it is that I have to try to make ends meet," she continued.

My heart went out to her. Life is just so unfair at times. How I wished I was a woman of means. I'd bloody set up a fund to help people who find themselves in similar circumstances.

Not long after, my name was called.

"I'll hopefully see you again," I told this woman, as I sympathetically gave her a gentle rub on the shoulder.

I was like an excited child on the morning of my very last treatment of radiotherapy.

"Just think; the very last time I will have to walk through the doors of the radiotherapy department," I told John.

I couldn't wait to get it over with, as I found myself rushing John in the hope that if I arrived at the department early, I would also be seen early. Once there, I beamed from ear to ear, almost as if to say to everyone that crossed my path, "That's me; I've done it! I have reached the last hurdle in my long battle to survive."

Almost a year of my life had been taken from me and put in the hands of others. Now it was time for me to take it back.

Chapter Twenty-One

Hi, My Name's Roseann

With all of my treatments complete and having started my drug therapy of Tamoxifen, all that was left for me to do now was focus on regaining my strength. I felt elated knowing that I now had my life back.

Throughout the year that followed, I took each day at a time and slowly, but gradually, I returned to the person that I once was and more. My experiences of having cancer and my road to recovery had given me a whole new hunger for life. I now wanted to take the time to really look at what was around me. I felt as if I had been reborn. My attitude and outlook on life had changed so much. On re-evaluating the important things in my life, I was amazed by how different they had now become. I now wanted to enjoy the simple things we take so much for granted, like that great gasp of breath you inhale on a windy day, or watching my garden change through the seasons. These simple pleasures uplifted me in a way I had never known before. It was almost as though someone had removed a pair of invisible blinkers from my eyes.

My family values had now become the most important thing in my life; I felt I was now able to see much more of the individual that was in each member of my family, something that I had never before noticed and most probably wouldn't have if I had not been faced with death. It was great to be alive again and I loved every minute of it.

As the months passed, I gradually grew more confident, finding that as I got stronger so did my self-esteem. Less frequently did I experience those long bouts of everlasting tears, the ones that would be accompanied by an array of morbid thoughts and raw emotions. Yes, I knew that there would always be a chance that my cancer could return, but I couldn't let these issues rule my life. I had a second chance and I was going to make the most of it.

Isabell had now stopped visiting on a regular basis. I can't really remember how that actually came about. There was no, "Well Roseann, this is the last time you will see me". Her visits just seemed to diminish gradually and the closeness we once shared seemed to become just a happy memory. I do, on very rare occasions, bump into her in the street or at the health centre and we always stop to say hello to each other, but as she walks away I always think of all the other people she visits now and find myself smiling, knowing just how fortunate they are, as was I, to have such a wonderful person touch our lives.

My ties with Marie my physiotherapist had also been severed; there was no need for me to visit her any longer now that my arm had regained almost the entire range of movements that it had before my surgery. It was such an amazing achievement when I think back to just how restricted and non-functional it was on the first day of my physiotherapy regime. Saying my goodbyes to Marie was really quite emotional. I had so much to be thankful to her for. Without her help, I knew that I would never have had the strength to get through the pain barriers I had to experience, caused by the stretching of an extremely seized up arm and shortened tendons. At times it felt as though someone had placed a very tight elastic band inside my arm and when Marie stretched it the pain could be unbearable. Many a time I had to tell her to stop in order to catch my breath. But that was all behind me now. It was time to turn another page in my book of life and move on.

With now two of my very important safety nets gone, I was surprised that I didn't feel as vulnerable as I thought I might. Funny how at one stage in my life I could never imagine being able to cope without people like Marie or Isabell, yet here I was standing once again on my own two feet.

In June of 2001, John and I excitedly prepared to go on a much needed holiday abroad, something that I had not been allowed to do for the past 17 months. We looked upon it as both my 40th birthday present and our anniversary present all rolled up into one. We holidayed in Cyprus and had the most amazing time. It was wonderful to feel the sun on my face and enjoy the fantastic scenery. We would spend endless hours sitting in an upper open lounge of one of the local bars watching all the younger holiday makers enjoy their nights on the town, their laughter filling the air. We even booked a mini cruise to Egypt to see the pyramids, something John had always dreamed of but never thought he would achieve.

On our return to Cyprus from Egypt, John and I were wandering around the local town where we stayed, lazily enjoying its peaceful atmosphere. Passing a jeweller's shop, I felt instantly drawn to it and pulled John over so I could look in the window. I could hardly believe my eyes as there staring me right in the face was the most gorgeous diamond ring I had ever seen.

"Come on, let me buy it for your birthday," John said.

It was at that moment, for the first time since my diagnosis of breast cancer, that I instantly believed that I would be that grey-haired old woman who in many years to come would look at that grey-haired old man and reminisce about how we had bought this beautiful token of love.

I felt a million dollars leaving the jeweller's with that ring, not in its box but snugly sitting next to my wedding ring on my left hand, glimmering in the light of the day. It was truly a memorable moment in my life that I will never forget. It sure felt good to be alive.

I am glad to say as I sit here talking with you that I have now been cancer free for 10 years. I focus only on living and now eagerly pursue my dreams. I have no time to die; there are still too many things in life that I have yet achieve.

My dream to visit Las Vegas? Yes, I did make the trip and even flew by helicopter into the Grand Canyon; an amazing experience.

I Am Not Alone

I know of individuals like me who have once again been given the gift of life; people that I would not otherwise have had the privilege of knowing, nor of hearing their very personal and intimate stories shared through the opening of hearts by one cancer sufferer to another.

Often the link between professionals and the cancer patient is broken on the conclusion of treatments. Not only do patients lose contact with their exceptionally skilled medical teams, but also with many people who have shared a short part of their lives; people who, like me, continue successfully along the road of life.

There are many accomplished stories out there of people who have fought and won their own very personal battles against cancer of all types.

Sheila: To have survived and lived a full and happy 20 years, after winning her own personal fight against breast cancer.

Peter: To have successfully made a full recovery after been diagnosed with testicular cancer and after surgery and subsequent treatments.

Lisa: To have battled ovarian cancer, endured surgery and invasive treatments and now to be living her life as she once did, cancer free.

Just a few success stories that prove how advancement and development in treatments, as Professor Cooke mentioned, has radically increased survival rates.

We rarely talk or hear of these others than via close knit family or local community settings and at times and I know that had I not suffered from cancer myself, I would most probably not have given success stories a second thought, other than a singular battle having being won via a short media acknowledgement.

Why? I believe that it is human nature not to feel the need to read statistical data on improvements in life expectancies associated with this terrible disease until it touches us on a personal level.

To all of you out there who passionately and tirelessly dedicate so much of your lives to supporting cancer organisations, charities, hospitals and specialised care facilities, I thank you, as without your support so many amazing feats could never have – nor ever will be – achieved.

Epilogue

Sadly, life can be cruel and just when we feel we have faced the biggest challenge we will ever have to endure in our lives, fate takes another turn by reminding us just how fragile the gift of life truly is.

My dream of being that grey-haired old lady living a wonderful life with that grey-haired old man was tragically shattered by the sudden death of my wonderful husband and soul mate on 22 January 2009 due to a massive heart attack at the age of just 46 years.

Another story that needs to be told … .